ANTI INFLAMMATORY MEAL PLAN

Simple And Easy Recipes Guide For Healing And Wellness

LISA BROWN

CONTENTS

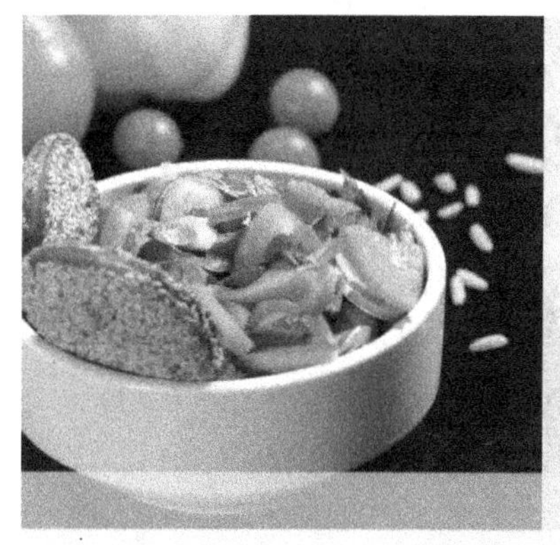
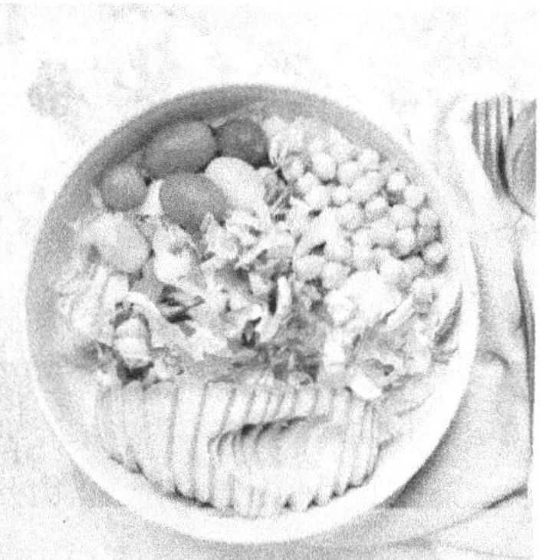

ANTI INFLAMMATORY MEAL PLAN

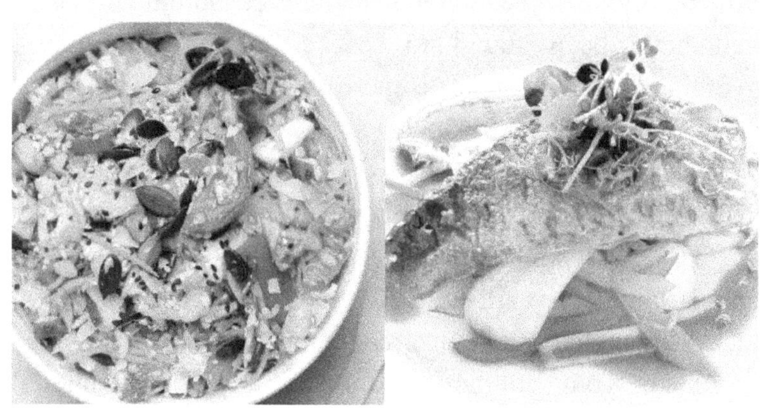

INTRODUCTION

The anti-inflammatory diet emphasizes complex carbs, legumes, nutrient-dense meals, healthy fats, and an abundance of fruits and vegetables. Red meat, processed meals, refined carbohydrates (such as white bread and white flour), and too much added sugar will not be seen more than once or twice a week. Reducing the body's chronic inflammation is the aim of this nutritious diet.

Despite the fact that inflammation is the body's natural response to acute injury, research links chronic inflammation to a number of chronic diseases, including diabetes, cancer, cardiovascular disease, nonalcoholic fatty liver disease, chronic kidney disease, autoimmune disorders, and neurodegenerative disorders.

By altering your lifestyle, you may reduce some of the inflammation. Some of them include consuming foods that have been found to reduce inflammation and avoiding those that tend to increase it, getting adequate sleep, exercising, and reducing stress.

This book is more than simply a compilation of recipes; it is a comprehensive guide to living an anti-inflammatory lifestyle. There are science-backed tactics, realistic meal plans, and simple-to-make recipes to make your journey stress-free and sustainable, regardless of whether you're battling certain health issues or just want to feel your best.

You will discover how to prepare meals efficiently, produce delicious foods that satisfy your hunger without compromising taste, and fill your pantry with anti-inflammatory staples. You can take charge of your health, beginning in your kitchen, with Anti-Inflammatory Diet Plan Prep's practical advice and easy-to-follow instructions.

Learn how eating the correct foods may increase general vitality, enhance digestion, and lessen inflammation. Regardless of your level of culinary expertise, this book provides all the information you need to adopt a way of life that puts enjoyment, healing, and health first. Take this as the first step to living a life free of inflammation and health.

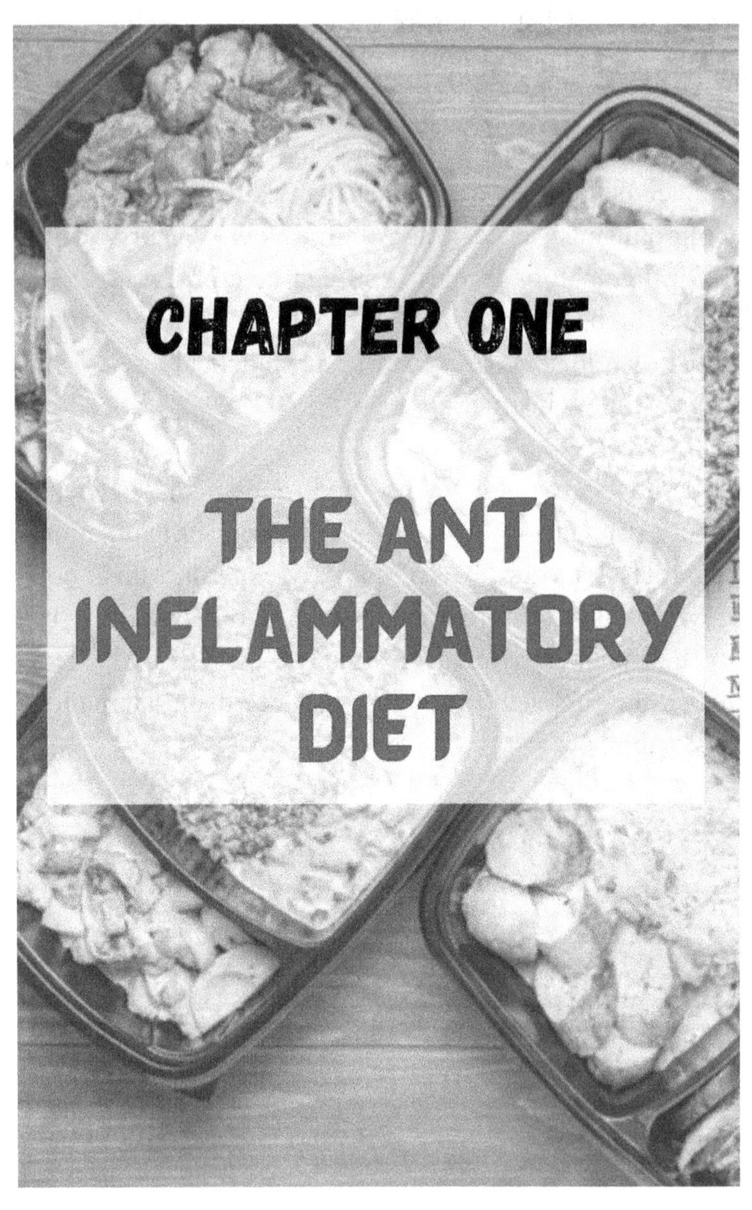
CHAPTER ONE

THE ANTI
INFLAMMATORY
DIET

CHAPTER 1

THE ANTI INFLAMMATORY DIET

Fresh fruits and vegetables, which are often excellent providers of antioxidants, are the mainstay of an anti-inflammatory diet.

Food compounds known as dietary antioxidants aid in the body's elimination of free radicals.

Naturally occurring byproducts of several body functions, such as metabolism, are free radicals. Cell damage may result from free radicals. This damage may lead to a number of disorders and raise the risk of inflammation.

Antioxidant-rich foods are preferred over those that increase the formation of free radicals in an anti-inflammatory diet.

Oily fish contains omega-3 fatty acids, which may help lower the body's levels of inflammatory proteins. Fiber can do the same thing.

Many illnesses that worsen with chronic inflammation may benefit from an anti-inflammatory diet as a supplemental treatment.

Inflammation is a factor in the following conditions:

- Psoriasis, asthma, and rheumatoid arthritis
- Esophagitis
- Crohn's disease
- IBD, or inflammatory bowel disease, includes colitis.
- Lupus
- Type 2 diabetes, Hashimoto's thyroiditis, and obesity
- High blood pressure
- Heart-related conditions.

Consuming a diet high in antioxidants may also help lower the chance of developing certain types of cancer.

Most Preferred Food To Eat

A diet that reduces inflammation should include a range of foods that:

- are abundant in nutrients.
- provide a variety of antioxidants and include good lipids.

The following foods may assist in the management of inflammation:

- fruits with rich colors, such as cherries, pomegranates, raspberries, and blueberries.

- leafy greens, such as spinach and kale.
- Cruciferous vegetables include cabbage, Brussels sprouts, cauliflower, and broccoli.
- entire grains that have not been refined, such as quinoa, barley, brown rice, or oats.
- legumes such as kidney, pinto, black, chickpeas, or lentils.
- Seeds and nuts.
- Avocados with olive oil.
- oily fish, such as mackerel, sardines, or salmon.
- Unsweetened black or green tea.
- dark chocolate.
- spices and herbs, including cinnamon, ginger, garlic, and turmeric.

It's important to keep in mind that no one meal will improve someone's health. A diverse range of nutritious foods should be included in the diet.

Limiting Foods:

When on an anti-inflammatory diet, people should minimize or stay away from:

- processed foods
- dishes with unhealthy oils or extra sugar or salt
- White bread, white spaghetti, and a variety of other baked items include processed carbohydrates.

- prepared snacks, such as crackers and chips
- prepared sweets, including ice cream, cookies, and candies
- Too much booze

Additionally, some individuals may be intolerant to certain foods, which means that consuming them may result in negative side effects like inflammation. Typical intolerances consist of:

- Dairy nightshade veggies that contain gluten
- Cruciferous veggies

Dietary advice for reducing inflammation

1. Switching to a new diet might be difficult, but the following advice could be useful:

2. During the weekly shop, pick up a range of fruits, vegetables, and nutritious snacks.

3. Replace fast food dinners with homemade, nutritious lunches over time.

4. Use still or sparkling mineral water in lieu of soda and other sugary drinks.

Other pointers are as follows:

- Discussing supplements, such as multivitamins or cod liver oil, with a medical expert.
- Integrating moderate exercise for 30 minutes each day into the schedule.
- Maintaining proper sleep hygiene since insufficient sleep exacerbates inflammation

SHOPPING LIST

PROTEINS
- black beans.
- kidney beans.
- Chickpeas.
- Lentils.
- Tofu.
- Tempeh.
- cottage cheese.
- Greek yogurt.
- seafood high in fat, like tuna or salmon.
- Chicken.
- Turkey.

CARBOHYDRATE
- whole oats.
- Whole wheat bread.
- Pasta made from whole wheat.
- Buckwheat.

- Cracked wheat, or bulgur.
- Farro.
- Barley.
- Freekeh.
- Quinoa.
- Rice.
- Millet.
- Amaranth.

VEGETABLES

- Tomatoes.
- Leafy greens, including spinach and kale.
- Sweet potatoes.
- Broccoli.
- Brussels sprouts.
- Cauliflower.
- Beets.
- Asparagus.
- Eggplant.
- Carrots.
- Bell peppers.
- Pumpkin.

FRUITS

- Strawberries.
- Blackberries.

- Cranberries.
- Blueberries.
- Apples.
- Pears.
- Cherries.
- Peaches.
- Apricots.
- plums.
- Grapes.
- Oranges.
- Grapefruit.
- Pomegranates.
- Avocado.

GOOD FATS

- Nuts like walnuts and almonds that aren't salted.
- Seeds that have not been salted, such as pumpkin and sunflower seeds.
- Seeds of chia.
- Flax seeds.
- Olive oil that is extra virgin.
- Avocado oil.
- Walnut oil.
- Hemp oil.
- Oil from flaxseed.

Additional anti-inflammatory, healthful pantry staples:

- Turmeric.
- Ginger.
- Powdered chili.
- Powdered garlic.
- Black pepper.
- Oregano.
- Thyme.
- Parsley.
- Rosemary.
- Sage.
- Canned tomatoes.
- Canned salmon or tuna.
- Potatoes.
- Onions.
- Pasta made from whole wheat.
- Canned beans.
- Oats rolled

ANTI-INFLAMMATORY DIETS BENEFITS

Anti-inflammatory foods are high in antioxidants, omega-3 fats, vitamins, minerals, and other healthy substances. Your immune system will function more effectively if you take these nutrients. An anti-inflammatory diet also prevents damaging inflammatory pathways throughout your body and protects your cells from injury.

The majority of chronic illnesses are less likely to strike those who follow anti-inflammatory diets. You may prevent the worsening of a chronic disease by following an anti-inflammatory diet. It could also assist you in controlling the symptoms of that long-term illness.

Numerous health advantages of an anti-inflammatory diet include:

Decreased risk of chronic illness: Eating a diet low in inflammation may help lower the chance of developing long-term conditions, including cancer, heart disease, and cognitive decline.

Better mental health: Eating a diet low in inflammation may improve mental and cognitive health.

Weight management: By increasing your sense of fullness while consuming fewer calories, an anti-inflammatory diet may assist you in maintaining a healthy weight.

Reduced symptoms: An anti-inflammatory diet may help reduce the symptoms of long-term illnesses such as lupus, arthritis, and inflammatory bowel disease.

Improved blood pressure: Eating a diet that reduces inflammation may help decrease blood pressure.

Increased levels of triglycerides, cholesterol, and blood sugar: An anti-inflammatory diet may contribute to an increase in these levels.

Enhanced vitality: Eating a diet low in inflammation might help boost vitality.

CHAPTER TWO

ANTI INFLAMMATORY MEAL PREP ESSENTIALS

- food to eat
- food to avoid
- meal prep tips

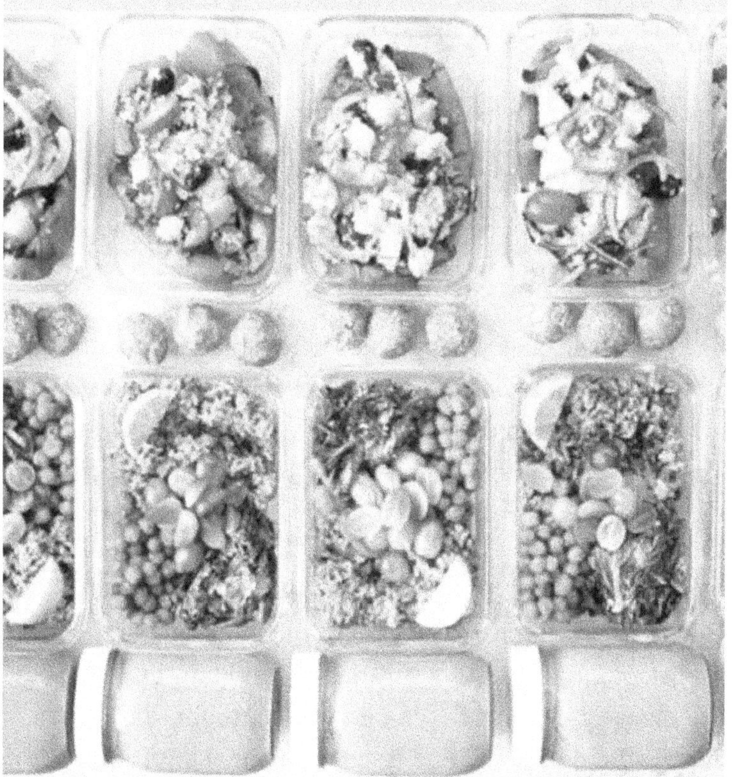

CHAPTER 2

MEAL PREP ESSENTIALS

There are several forms of meal preparation to take into account. While some individuals choose to cook just for the next week and keep the food in the refrigerator to reheat when needed, others prepare meals to freeze for a time when they don't have time to cook. Various forms of meal preparation consist of:

Make-ahead meals: these are dishes, like curries, that are prepared in advance and then frozen or refrigerated in portions. You can just thaw and reheat the meal when you're ready to consume it, eliminating the need for further preparation.

Batch cooking is the process of preparing a large amount of food in advance and storing it in the refrigerator or freezer for later use. In batch cooking, you may prepare four times the amount called for, freezing the other three portions and reserving one for later that night.

Ready-to-cook ingredients are those that have been prepared in advance for a particular dish, saving time when cooking later. For instance, chopping and peeling all the veggies for a casserole the night before and putting them in the fridge to cook the next day.

IDEAL MEAL PREP FOODS

Breakfasts, lunches, and dinners may all be prepared ahead of time, and there aren't many restrictions on what ingredients can and cannot be used for meal preparation.

The following foods are ideal for meal prep:

Fresh and frozen vegetables are included. All kinds of vegetables and salad elements may be cleaned, peeled, chopped, and cooked in advance.

Meat, fish, poultry, and vegetarian and vegan substitutes are examples of proteins. All protein components may be prepared ahead of time and then chilled so they are ready to consume.

Pasta, rice, couscous, beans, chickpeas, quinoa, and other pulses, grains, and carbs. These components often make up the majority of your meal prep meals and may all be prepared in advance.

Fruits: You may wash, peel, and cut any kind of fruit, then store it in the refrigerator or freezer.

Eggs: eggs may be prepared in advance by boiling or scrambling them, then reheated or consumed cold. Fried or poached eggs may also be prepared in advance, but they may not have the same texture when reheated, so you might choose to cook them fresh.

Duration for Meal Prep

Your prepared foods will last five days in the fridge or four months in the freezer if properly stored and cooled.

To prevent foodborne infections, it's critical to properly chill, store, and label your food after cooking. This entails chilling your prepared meals as soon as possible and avoiding the dangerous temperature range of 8 to 60 degrees Celsius. The likelihood of dangerous germs developing decreases with decreasing temperature.

Decant your prepared meals into appropriate containers when they have cooled, and mark them with the contents, the date of preparation, and the expiration date.

Using the proper storage containers can help extend the shelf life of your meals. Regardless of whether you decide to utilize glass jars, stainless steel tubs, reusable silicone bags, or plastic boxes, it's critical that your meal prep storage is:

- airtight and sealable.
- freezer-safe.
- impervious to leaks.

Is Preparing Meals Safe?

A crucial component of meal planning is food safety and cleanliness, as you must make sure the food you're making is free of dangerous microorganisms that may make you sick. Overall, meal planning is a safe method of food preparation; but, as you prepare, cook, chill, and store your prepared meals, observe these food safety guidelines:

- Before preparing, carefully wash your fruits and vegetables under running water to get rid of any dirt or debris that may have gotten on them.
- Hands should be thoroughly cleaned both before and after handling high-risk foods like raw fish and meat.
- Food must achieve at least 70 °C for two minutes, 75 °C for thirty seconds, or 80 °C for six seconds. Keep in mind these essential cooking temperatures. You may obtain this reading with the use of a probe thermometer.
- After cooking, try to bring food down to refrigerator temperature within 90 minutes.
- Maintain your refrigerator at 8 oC or lower. To stop germs from growing on food, it is best to keep it around 5 oC.
- For proper food hygiene, make sure you're keeping food on the appropriate refrigerator shelves.

- Defrost your freezer often and keep it set at -18 °C.
- Eat the defrosted food within 24 hours of it being securely thawed in the refrigerator rather than at room temperature.
- Reheating your prepared meals more than once raises the danger of food illness, so only do it once.

TIPS FOR MEAL PREP

The top ten meal prep suggestions listed below will help you maximize your cooking if you're new to meal prep:

Before you start cooking, compile a shopping list of all the items you'll need to make everything and then create a meal plan for the next week or month.

Now is the time to go through your recipe books, phone notes, or Pinterest meal ideas for inspiration, whether you want to try new dishes or stick to your old favorites. Do you want to prepare familiar and beloved foods or use this as a chance to try something different?

Choose a meal prep day. Professional meal preppers follow a pattern to help them remain on top of their meal prep, but it may be a Sunday afternoon activity or something you do every Monday night.

Decide which meals you want to prepare. Will you prepare meals for morning, noon, or dinner? Preparing meals that you often find difficult or typically lack the time to cook, like breakfast before the school run, might be beneficial.

To what extent will you prepare meals? Are you preparing meals for the next day, the upcoming week, or the whole month?

Prepare snacks and sweets in advance of meals. Having delights on hand might help you avoid impulsive purchases or unhealthy munching.

Make sure you have extra containers for storage. Make sure you have the right bags and tubs before you begin dinner prep; otherwise, you'll be left with a skillet full of food and nowhere to put it.

Take advantage of meal preparation as a chance to eat more nutrients. If you often have trouble eating properly, utilize meal prep to include more nutritionally balanced items into your diet and make veggies the main ingredient in your cooking.

Use your air fryer or slow cooker. You may save even more time and power by using these little electrical devices. You may use your air fryer for individual ingredients or your slow cooker for whole meals, such as casseroles and curries.

By ensuring that your food is already portioned out into separate, appropriate-sized amounts, meal prep may help you stay on top of portion management.

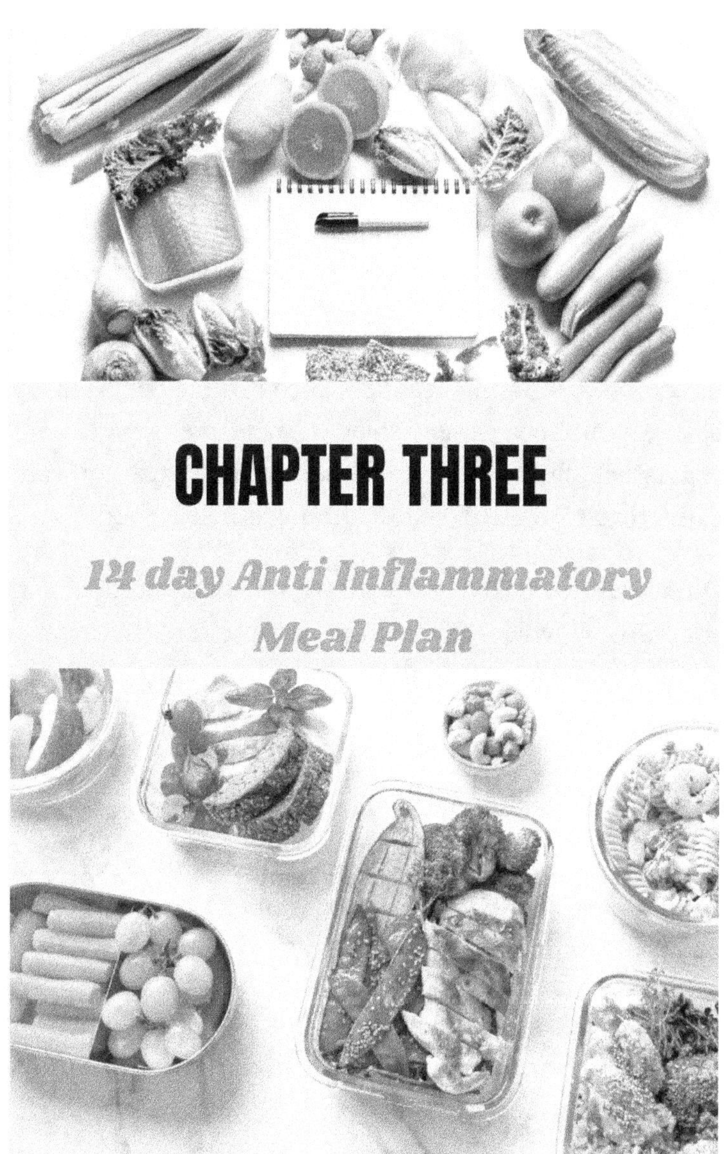

CHAPTER THREE

14 day Anti Inflammatory Meal Plan

CHAPTER 3

TWO WEEKS MEAL PREP PLAN

Day 1 Breakfast: Ground flaxseeds, cinnamon, blueberries, 1% milk (a low-fat dairy substitute), and honey drizzled over microwaved porridge.

Lunch: Low-sodium canned diced tomatoes, kidney beans, pinto beans, and black beans are served with vegetarian chili cooked without adding sugar or salt. Cornbread made with healthy grains is also served.

Dinner will be baked fish with fresh lemon juice, pepper, and garlic powder. Serve with your preferred seasoning on the asparagus and roasted carrots.

Snacks: Raw bell peppers with hummus, sliced apples, and air-popped popcorn.

Day 2 Breakfast: On hectic mornings, utilize leftovers from supper for breakfast for a quick, satisfying, and wholesome start to the day.

Lunch consists of roasted peppers seasoned with chili powder and garlic, black beans, and corn on top of a huge baked sweet potato.

If desired, top with a protein source, such as low-fat shredded cheese.

Dinner will be roasted chicken breast on a sheet pan with broccoli, cauliflower, onions, peppers, and Brussels sprouts. Add paprika, pepper, and garlic powder for seasoning. For dessert, garnish with fresh blackberries.

Snacks include grapes, almonds, and unsalted walnuts; cucumber slices with hummus.

Day 3 Breakfast: egg scramble with sautéed veggies and one egg. Serve with low-sodium peanut butter or nut butter and whole-grain bread.

Lunch consists of whole-grain rice with leftover sheet-pan roasted chicken and veggies.

Dinner is a simple loaded salad made with canned tuna in water, almonds, pepitas, tomatoes, cucumbers, and feta cheese on top of kale and spinach. Top with a drizzle of olive oil dressing. Serve with toast or whole grain crackers.

Snacks: Clementine and hard-boiled egg; almonds and unsweetened nonfat yogurt.

Day 4 Breakfast: Chia seeds, cinnamon, vanilla essence, 1% milk, or a dairy substitute are combined to make an overnight pudding. Add your preferred fruit on top.

Lunch is a whole-grain wrap with leftover salad, blackberries, and Greek yogurt.

Dinner is either chickpea noodles or whole-wheat noodles with a spaghetti sauce prepared with ground chicken, chopped tomatoes, mushrooms, garlic powder, and oregano. Serve with roasted green beans.

Snacks include carrot sticks, Brazil nuts, edamame, and a little apple.

Day 5 Breakfast: A smoothie consisting of 1% milk or a dairy substitute, spinach, banana, blueberries, and kefir. Ground flaxseeds or chia seeds may be added. Serve with black coffee.

Lunch is leftover noodles and spaghetti. Serve with tiny carrots on the side.

Dinner will be chicken tortilla soup with limes, cumin, garlic, corn, black beans, tomatoes, and onions.

served with fresh salsa and whole-grain cornbread.

Snacks include chopped veggies with vinaigrette dressing and an apple with melted nut butter.

Day 6 Breakfast: Whole-grain bread with a pear or other fruit of your choosing on the side and half of an avocado on top.

Lunch consists of corn tortillas, salsa, and leftover chicken tortilla soup.

Dinner will be steamed broccoli and roasted sweet potatoes accompanied with air-fried fish. When baking or air-frying sweet potatoes, use olive oil.

Snacks: energy bites and carrot sticks with red pepper hummus.

Day 7 Breakfast: Overnight oats are prepared with traditional oats, chia seeds, your favorite milk, honey or maple syrup, and a dash of salt. For a more substantial breakfast, you may also mix in some plain low-fat Greek yogurt for extra protein.

Lunch is a Green Goddess sandwich with broccoli sprouts, spinach, sliced avocados, cucumber, and whole-grain bread.

Add lemon juice, parsley, chives, tarragon, garlic, and a Greek yogurt dressing over top.

Dinner: Curry powder, ginger, garlic, turmeric, spinach, coconut milk, red peppers, tomatoes, cauliflower, and a chicken and chickpea curry stuffed with vegetables.

Snacks include unsweetened dry fruit, pumpkin seeds, and broccoli with Greek yogurt ranch dip.

Day 8 breakfast: Smoothie prepared with a combination of berries, frozen riced cauliflower, kefir, 1% milk or a dairy substitute, almonds, chia, or ground flaxseeds for breakfast on day eight. Serve with black coffee.

Lunch is a leftover curry made with chicken and chickpeas and laden with vegetables. If preferred, serve with whole-grain naan.

Dinner will be a salmon rice bowl with diced avocado on top of brown rice, cabbage, cucumbers, and green onions.

Snacks: dried figs, almonds, a little piece of dark chocolate, oranges, and low-fat cottage cheese.

Day 9 Breakfast: Blueberries and sliced almonds on top of low-sugar, nonfat Greek yogurt. Hot coffee with 1% milk added.

Lunch is a leftover salmon rice dish, which tastes delicious cold if you dislike the scent of warmed fish. Serve with fruit.

Dinner is a spinach salad with balsamic dressing, roasted butternut squash, blueberries, quinoa, figs, and red onions on top.

Snacks: carrots with Greek yogurt ranch dip and cumin-seasoned roasted chickpeas.

Day 10 Breakfast: A whole-grain tortilla wrapped in a breakfast burrito with sautéed black beans, tomatoes, and peppers.

Serve with a dollop of low-fat shredded cheese and salsa.

Lunch is a chickpea salad sandwich with tomatoes, lettuce, red onion, celery, garlic, lemon juice, and olive oil. Accompany the dish with carrots and berries.

Dinner will be baked tilapia accompanied by butternut squash and leftover spinach salad with figs.

Snacks include dark chocolate, walnuts, figs, and peanut butter on whole-grain bread.

Day 11 Breakfast: Premade energy bites made with crushed flax seed, low-sodium nut or seed butter, vanilla extract, honey, unsweetened dried fruit, and old-fashioned oats. Serve with your preferred fruit, such as berries, bananas, or apples.

Lunch is a cold lentil salad dressed with olive oil vinaigrette and composed of cucumber, feta cheese, tomatoes, and olives. Serve with carrots and hummus.

Dinner is a sweet potato hash with ground turkey, cumin, garlic powder, chopped tomatoes, peppers, and chiles.

Snacks include whole-grain crackers, low-fat cheese, and popcorn dusted with cinnamon.

Day 12 Breakfast: Whole-grain bread with peppers, spinach, mushrooms, and a scrambled egg on top. Accompany the dish with fresh strawberries.

Lunch will be sweet potato hash leftovers. On the side, place a clementine.

Dinner will be potatoes and lemon garlic chicken in a single pan. Serve with your preferred green veggies, such as asparagus, broccoli, or green beans.

Snacks include a piece of low-fat cheese, a peach, and chia pudding with cinnamon and vanilla.

Day 13 Breakfast: A smoothie prepared with 1% milk, unsweetened kefir, or a dairy substitute.

Add chia seeds, unsweetened cocoa powder, low-sodium nut or seed butter, and a medium banana. Enjoy with a cup of black coffee!

Lunch consists of potatoes, veggies, and leftover lemon garlic chicken.

Dinner will be roasted sweet potatoes stuffed with chickpeas seasoned with the southwest, tomatoes, onions, and garlic.

Snacks: hummus, peppers, carrots, and energy bites.

Day 14 Breakfast: Whole-grain bread with a banana slice, a handful of almonds, and low-sodium butternut on top. Enjoy with a cup of black coffee!

Lunch is leftover sweet potatoes with a southwest filling.

Dinner consists of toasted corn tortillas stuffed with salmon on tacos and a creamy avocado-lime broccoli salad.

Snacks: Greek yogurt and almonds; blueberries and walnuts.

LIFESTYLE CHANGES FOR AN ANTI INFLAMMATORY LIFESTYLE

By adopting these lifestyle modifications, you can lower chronic inflammation:

Consume foods that reduce inflammation: Antioxidants, flavonoids, and omega-3 fatty acids are found in diets that reduce inflammation. These consist of cruciferous vegetables (broccoli, cauliflower, and

Brussels sprouts), leafy greens (arugula, spinach, and kale), fatty fish (salmon, tuna, and mackerel), nuts and seeds (almonds, flaxseed, and chia seeds), fruits (mangoes, oranges, berries, apples, and berries), olive oil, curcumin (found in turmeric), green tea, and black tea.

Give up smoking.: See your primary care physician about quitting smoking, vaping, or using tobacco products.

Avoid or limit alcohol: Limit or stay away from alcoholic drinks if you wish to reduce inflammation.

Steer clear of foods that cause inflammation. Reduce your consumption of red and processed meats (such as beef, pork, lamb, bacon, sausage, and salami), fried foods, refined carbohydrates (such as white pasta, bread, and rice), dairy, and processed foods (such as chips, crackers, and freezer meals). Sugar is frequently present in desserts, candy, baked goods, soda, fruit juice, and even ketchup and pasta sauce.

Use stress-reduction strategies: Make time for stress-relieving pursuits like yoga, journaling, meditation, nature walks, reading, gardening, or other hobbies since stress may cause inflammation in the body. Take a break from using your computer, phone, and other electronics to relax, reflect, and work through your emotions.

Keep your weight in check: Find out from your primary care physician whether your weight is appropriate for your height, age, and other characteristics. Inquire with your healthcare professional about the safest and healthiest methods of losing weight if you are overweight or obese.

Engage in regular exercise: Maintaining a healthy weight, reducing stress, improving digestion, and maintaining strong bones and muscular mass are all made possible by regular exercise. Aim for 150 minutes of moderate cardiovascular exercise each week, such as walking, bicycling, swimming, hiking, tennis, dancing, or aerobics, in addition to at least two strength training sessions.

Maintain proper sleep hygiene: Try to sleep seven to nine hours every night, avoid using electronics an hour before bed, buy a comfortable mattress, pillow, and sheets, use a white noise machine to drown out distractions, sleep in a cool, dark room, and see your primary care physician if you experience fatigue frequently.

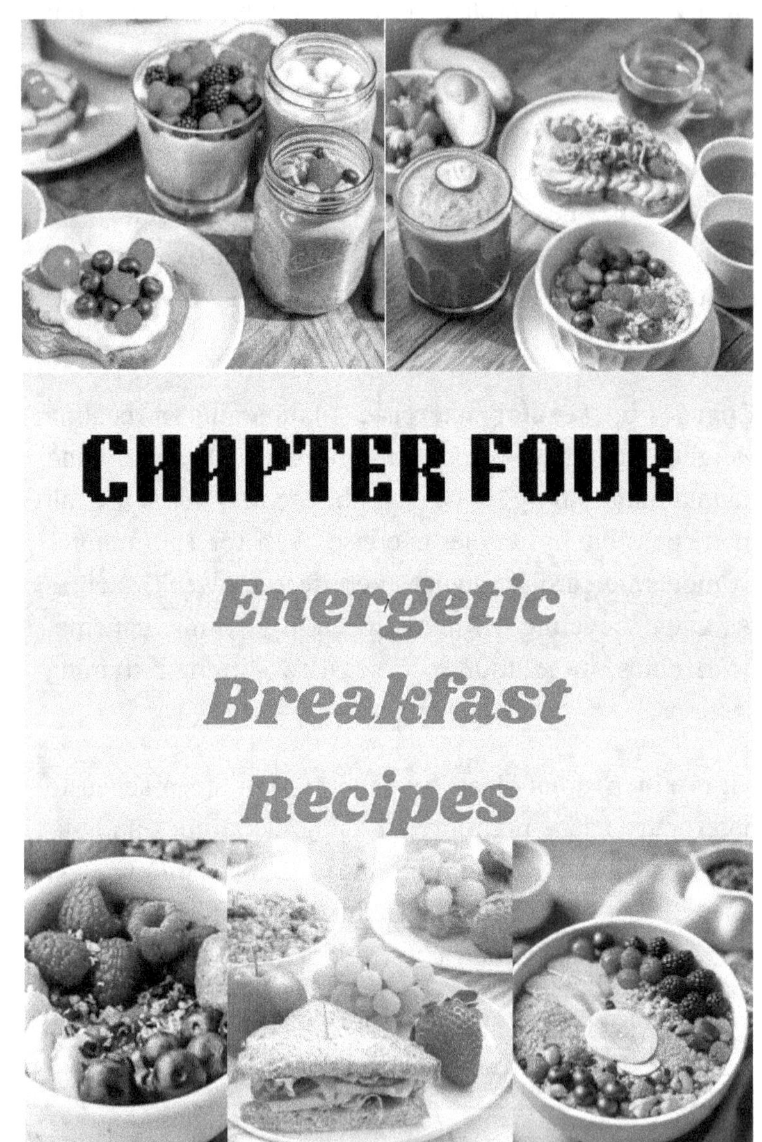

CHAPTER FOUR

Energetic Breakfast Recipes

CHAPTER 4

BREAKFAST RECIPES

Super Greens Powder Smoothie

Ingredients

- One cup of pineapple, frozen
- One cup of frozen bananas or mangoes
- One spoonful of powdered super greens
- Half a cup of full-fat yogurt
- 1½ cups of coconut water without sugar
- Chia Pudding with Powdered Super Greens
- Two tablespoons of chia seeds
- One spoonful of powdered super greens
- Half a cup of coconut milk

Instructions

1. Put all the ingredients for the super green smoothie in your blender.
2. One cup of frozen mango or banana, one cup of frozen pineapple, one tablespoon of super greens powder, half a cup of whole milk yogurt, and half a cup of unsweetened coconut water

3. Blend your smoothie until the frozen fruit is all gone.
4. Transfer to a glass and savor!

Parfait with Fruit and Herbs

Ingredients:

- ¾ cup Greek-style yogurt with reduced fat
- ⅓ cup of fresh fruit, diced (we garnished with pieces of star fruit, mandarin segments, bananas, kiwis, strawberries, and rockmelon).
- To garnish, add ⅓ cup of oats and fresh mint leaves.
- One teaspoon of goji or freeze-dried raspberries, if desired, as a garnish.

Instructions

1. Place half the Greek-style yogurt, half the granola, and half of the chopped fruit in a small glass or jar.
2. Repeat and, if using, garnish with freeze-dried raspberries or goji and fresh mint.

Nutrition (per serving)

410 calories

Carbs: 1700 kJ

22 g of protein, 11 g of total fat

3.6 g of saturated fat, 48 g of carbohydrates

26 g of sugar, 8.5 g of dietary fiber

236 milligrams of sodium, 323 mg of calcium

Iron 0.5 mg

Walnut-Cinnamon Brown Rice Pudding

Ingredients

- Four cups of water
- One cup of brown rice
- Four cups of almond milk
- Two tablespoons of sugar
- Two tablespoons of honey
- One Tablespoon of cinnamon
- One teaspoon of nutmeg
- Two tablespoons of butter
- Half a cup of raisins

Instructions

1. Add the brown rice and bring 4 cups of water to a boil.
2. Reduce the heat to medium, cover the rice, and cook it for half an hour.

3. Stir from time to time. Return the rice to the pot after draining the water.
4. Remove the saucepan from the stove and let it steam for ten minutes.
5. Ten minutes later, move the rice to a bowl and put it away.
6. Bring sugar, honey, almond milk, and spices to a gentle boil.
7. To prevent the milk from burning, stir often.
8. Stir often after adding the rice, butter, and raisins.
9. Simmer for 30 to 45 minutes, or until the milk has cooked down.
10. Sprinkle some cinnamon on top and serve cold or room-temperature.

NUTRITION: per serving

6 servings

189 calories

6 g of total fat, 3 g of saturated fat

0g of trans fat, 3 g of unsaturated fat.

10 mg of cholesterol, 45 milligrams of sodium

34 g of carbohydrates, 2 g of fiber.

22 g of sugar, 2 g of protein.

Stovetop Steel-cut Oats With Almonds, Bananas, And Cherries

Ingredients:

- 1 cup steel-cut oats (gluten-free, if necessary) and 3 cups water
- a pinch of salt.
- 1/4 cup milk, plus more as needed (almond, cashew, banana, cherries, and coconut were used).
- Half a teaspoon of vanilla

Instructions

1. First, bring the water to a boil. In a medium saucepan over medium-high heat, bring the water to a boil.
2. Add salt and oats. Add the steel-cut oats and a little amount (less than 1/8 tsp.) of salt to the boiling water.
3. Stir and simmer. Lower the heat to low and cook for 15 to 20 minutes, or until the oatmeal is soft and most of the water has been absorbed.
4. Finish with a taste. After adding the milk and vanilla, turn it off here.

Nutrition: per serving

Four servings

Calories. 174 kcal

3%2.7g of total fat, 0.5g of saturated fat,

0% cholesterol, and 0 mg, 91.5 mg of 4% sodium

31.2g of total carbohydrates, 18% dietary fiber, 5g of sugars, 10%, and 5.1g of protein,

0%0 mg of vitamin C, 57.7 mg of calcium at 4%

1% Magnesium 3 mg

151.8 mg of 3% potassium

Coconut Flour Pancake

Ingredients:

- ¼ cup coconut flour (measure with a level)
- Three huge eggs
- Two teaspoons of olive oil
- Two teaspoons of maple syrup (or keto-friendly sugar-free syrup)
- (See remark) 1 teaspoon baking powder
- One teaspoon of vanilla extract
- ⅛ teaspoon of sea salt, fine

Instructions

1. The coconut flour, eggs, oil, baking powder, maple syrup, vanilla extract, and salt should all be combined in a big basin. Break up any clumps by stirring everything together with a whisk. (The batter will be considerably thicker and more difficult to work with if coconut oil is used.)
2. Put 2 tablespoons of the pancake mixture in an oiled skillet over medium-low heat and cook for approximately 4 minutes, or until bubbles begin to appear in the center of the pancake. After flipping, heat for a further 4 minutes or until the pancake is brown on both sides. The pancake's outside may burn before the inside is cooked through and fluffy, so resist the urge to turn up the heat to expedite the cooking process.
3. Make around five little pancakes (about 4 to 5 inches in diameter) by repeating with the remaining batter. Top with your preferred toppings and serve warm. Pancake leftovers may be kept in the refrigerator for up to five days in an airtight container.

Nutrition: per-serving

2 servings

343 kcal, 24 g of carbohydrates, 10 g of protein,

22 g of fat, 6 g of saturated fat,

3 g of polyunsaturated fat, 13 g of monounsaturated fat, 0.03 g of trans fat, 246 mg of cholesterol,

275 mg of sodium, 341 mg of potassium, 5 g of fiber, 14 g of sugar, 356 IU of vitamin A,

146 mg of calcium, and 2 mg of iron

Zucchini Breakfast Muffins

Ingredients

- Two whisked eggs
- 40 milliliters of frying oil
- Place the following in a bowl.
- Half a shredded carrot
- Half a cup of grated zucchini
- 30 grams of shredded cheese—I use cheddar.
- 60 grams of self-raising flour
- A dash of salt and pepper

Instructions

1. Set oven temperature to 180°C. Apply butter to seven of the muffin tin's holes.
2. To the bowl containing the flour, cheese, and vegetables, add the egg and oil combination. Mix thoroughly.
3. Fill each muffin hole with an equal amount of the mixture. Bake for 15 to 18 minutes, or until the

top is lightly golden brown. Let cool in muffin tin, then take out.

Chile-cumin Scrambled Eggs

Ingredients:

- two eggs
- Half a cup of chopped onion
- Half a cup of milk
- Two teaspoons of green bell pepper, chopped
- Two teaspoons of red bell pepper, chopped
- One chopped and seeded jalapeño pepper
- Two tablespoons of chili powder, Mexican style
- One teaspoon of powdered onion
- Half a teaspoon of cumin powder
- One dab of ground cinnamon
- To taste, add salt and ground black pepper.
- cooking spray.

Instructions

1. In a bowl, whisk eggs together. Add the onion, milk, bell peppers, cumin, cinnamon, salt, black pepper, chili powder, onion powder, and jalapeño pepper.
2. Apply cooking spray to a big skillet and heat it over medium-high heat. After adding the egg

mixture to the pan, heat and stir for about five minutes, or until golden brown.

Nutrition: per-serving

One serving

233 calories

16g Carbs, 16g Protein, and 12g Fat

Avocado And Egg Breakfast Sandwich

Ingredients

1. One tablespoon of olive oil
2. Two large eggs
3. To taste, add salt and ground black pepper.
4. One tablespoon of softened butter
5. Two pieces of Italian bread
6. One ounce of sliced Swiss cheese
7. One ounce of sliced cheddar cheese
8. Sliced ½ ripe avocado

Instructions

1. In a pan, heat the olive oil over medium heat. Add the eggs to the skillet and cook for one to two minutes. Cook the egg for another 2 to 5

minutes after flipping it. Add salt and pepper to the eggs after transferring them to a platter.

2. On one side of each piece of bread, spread butter. A skillet should be heated to medium heat. Place pieces of bread, butter side down, in the heated skillet. Quickly arrange the remaining piece of bread, butter-side up, followed by Swiss cheese, one fried egg, cheddar cheese, avocado, then another fried egg.

3. Flip the sandwich carefully to the opposite side of the grill and cook for 3 to 4 minutes, or until golden brown.

4. Slice the sandwich in half after taking it out of the griddle.

Nutrition:per-serving

One serving

552 calories

22g Carbs, 18g Protein, and 44g Fat

Berry And Chia Seed Pudding

Ingredients

- Two cups of milk
- Eight tablespoons Half a cup of chia seeds

- A half-cup of mixed berries Raspberry, blackberry, and blueberry
- Two tablespoons of honey or agave sweetener
- Half a teaspoon of vanilla

Instructions

1. In a blender, combine the milk, mixed berries, sugar, and vanilla; process until smooth.
2. The liquid should be split between two containers.
3. To each, add 4 tablespoons of chia seeds and stir them in.
4. Cover and let for 20 minutes, then stir one more.
5. Keep in the fridge for at least four hours, but ideally overnight.

Sweet Potato Hash

Ingredients

- 1.5 pounds of sweet potatoes (about two medium ones)
- One yellow onion
- One red bell pepper
- Breakfast sausage, 8 oz.
- Tbsp frying oil, half
- 3/4 teaspoon of salt
- Half a teaspoon of freshly ground black pepper

- A half-tsp of garlic powder
- Half a teaspoon smoked paprika

Instructions

1. Clean the sweet potatoes, peel them, and chop them. Chop the red bell pepper and onion. Place the veggies aside.

2. Crumble the morning sausage and sauté it over medium heat in a large nonstick pan. Sauté the sausage until it is almost browned. Continue heating after adding the chopped onion until it becomes transparent and the sausage has completely browned. Transfer the onions and sausage to a different platter and put them aside.

3. Add the frying oil and the chopped sweet potatoes to the same skillet. For ten to twelve minutes, cook the sweet potatoes over medium heat. To give the sweet potatoes time to brown and caramelize, stir them periodically but not too often. The sweet potatoes will continue to cook in the next stage, so don't worry if they are not fork-tender at this point.

4. Now add the smoked paprika, garlic powder, black pepper, salt, and chopped red bell pepper to the pan. Add the sweet potatoes and stir. Cook until the sweet potatoes are fork-tender, about 3 to 5 more minutes.

5. Return the cooked sausage and onions to the pan and mix them with the peppers and sweet potatoes. To enable the sausage to reheat with the remaining hash, cook for an additional one to two minutes.

6. Serve this sweet potato hash with sliced avocado, fresh parsley, or any toppings you choose!

Nutrition: per-serving

One serving

227 kcal of calories, 26g of carbohydrates, 8g of protein

10g of fat, 595 milligrams of sodium, 4g of fiber.

Tofu Scramble

Ingredients
- Two tablespoons of extra-virgin olive oil and one pound of extra-firm tofu
- Two sliced garlic cloves
- One sliced onion
- Curry powder, 2 1/2 tablespoons
- Two teaspoons of optional nutritional yeast
- Three large handfuls of stemmed spinach leaves
- Half a teaspoon of fine sea salt, plus more if necessary
- To serve: spicy sauce and chives

Instructions

1. After removing any remaining water, crush the tofu into tiny pieces and press them between two paper towels to remove any moisture.
2. Heat the oil in a big, heavy pan over medium heat, add the garlic and onion, and sauté for just a few minutes until they soften up. Add the tofu and curry powder and stir. Cover and simmer until the tofu is cooked through, about 4–5 minutes. Add the spinach and stir in the nutritional yeast. Add the salt after a minute or two of stirring, until it wilts and collapses. Adjust for seasoning by tasting. Add extra curry powder if you want the curry taste to be more vibrant. A few pinches of salt at a time may be added if the flavors aren't quite bursting.

Nutrition: per- serving

Calories 129 kcal , Fat 8g, Saturated Fat 1g
Polyunsaturated Fat 2g, Monounsaturated Fat 4g
Sodium 306mg
353 mg of potassium, 7g of carbohydrates, 2g of fiber, 2g of sugar, and 9g of protein
1698 IU of vitamin A and 7 mg of vitamin C
Iron 2 mg, calcium 58 mg

Breakfast Bowl with Quinoa

Ingredients

- 1 1/2 cups water and 3/4 cup dried quinoa

- 3/4 cup of coconut milk in a can
- Half a cup of nondairy milk, with more for garnish
- One chopped date or one tablespoon of optional maple syrup
- Two tablespoons of cinnamon powder
- Two tablespoons of vanilla extract
- A pinch of salt
- Whatever toppings you desire! (Chocolate chips, banana, blueberries, peanut butter, coconut flakes, walnuts, and chia seeds)

Instructions

1. In a medium saucepan, add quinoa and water. Bring to a boil, then lower the heat to a simmer, cover, and cook until the quinoa is frothy, 13 to 15 minutes.
2. Don't turn up the heat. Add salt, cinnamon, vanilla, sweetener, coconut milk, and nondairy milk. Mix to blend. Cook until the quinoa is still pouring but has absorbed most of the milk. If necessary, add more non-dairy milk.
3. Transfer some to a bowl and garnish with more nondairy milk and other desired toppings, such as nuts, fruit, or nut butter—the options are unlimited!

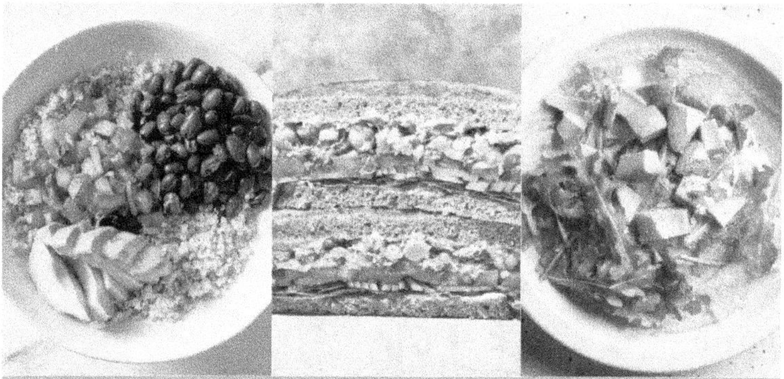

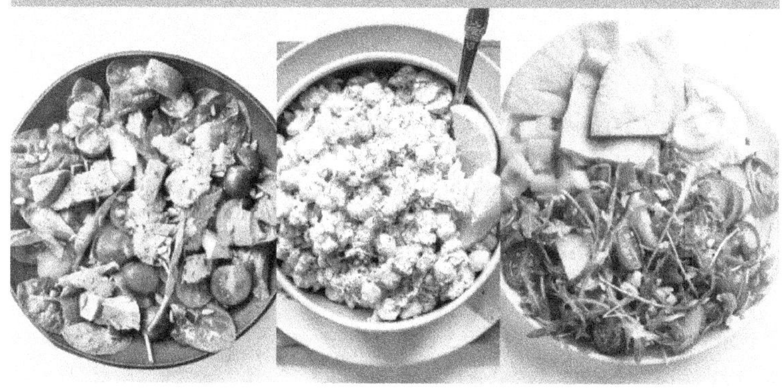

CHAPTER FIVE

DELICIOUS ANTI INFLAMMATORY DIET LUNCH IDEAS

CHAPTER 5

LUNCH RECIPES

Grill Salmon Salad

Ingredients

- Two cups of greens, such as baby spinach, mustard greens, lettuce, or baby arugula
- Five cherry tomatoes, cut in half
- 1/4 cup chopped red onions
- Half a cup of chopped cucumbers
- Half an avocado, chopped
- One or two teaspoons of vinegar
- One salmon filet, or around 4 ounces
- Half a teaspoon of olive oil
- To taste, add kosher salt.
- To taste, freshly ground black pepper

Instructions

1. Add the avocado, cucumbers, red onions, cherry tomatoes, and greens to a bowl. Pour some vinaigrette over it. Put aside.
2. Using the highest setting, preheat the grill to around 500 degrees.

3. Add salt and pepper to the fish after brushing it with olive oil.
4. Put the salmon on the grill and cook it for six minutes without moving it. Cook for a further four to five minutes after flipping, or until done. When it's done, the salmon should come out of the grills with ease.
5. Eat the salmon right away after placing it on the salad.

Nutrition: per-serving

440 calories

43 g of protein, 28 g of fat.

4g of saturated fat, 1.8g of omega-3 fatty acids

12 g of carbohydrates, 7g of fiber, 5 g of sugar.

Lentils and Vegetable Soup

Ingredients

- One yellow onion
- One big carrot (or two tiny) and two celery stalks
- Five ounces of mushrooms
- Eight ounces of white potato (about one medium)
- Four garlic cloves
- 15 oz. can of fire-roasted or diced tomatoes

- One cup of uncooked green or brown lentils and six glasses of vegetable broth
- 1 1/2 teaspoons of Italian spice
- One or two cups of fresh baby spinach, if desired

Instructions

1. Chop the celery, carrot, and onion. Dice the potatoes and mushrooms. Put aside.
2. Combine the celery, carrot, and onion in a stockpot and heat it at medium-high heat. Sauté for seven to eight minutes. (For the no-oil sauté technique, I use 3 tablespoons of water or vegetable broth; I add more as necessary.)
3. In the meantime, chop the garlic.
4. Add the garlic, mushrooms, potato, and Italian spice after the onion has become transparent. For two to three minutes, stir and sauté.
5. Add the rinsed and drained lentils, diced tomatoes, and vegetable broth. Raise the heat until it comes to a gentle boil.
6. After that, lower the heat, cover, and simmer the lentils gently for 25 to 30 minutes, or until they are soft.
7. In the last few minutes of cooking, add the roughly chopped spinach and toss it in. Season with salt and pepper.

Nutrition: per-serving

Total calories per serving: 190 kcal

1 g of fat, 0.1g of saturated fat

0.3g of polyunsaturated fat

0.1g of monounsaturated fat

809 milligrams of potassium

37 g of carbohydrates, 13 g of fiber.

7 g of sugar, 11g of protein

2833 IU of vitamin A, 20 mg of vitamin C

75 mg of calcium, 4 mg of iron

Quinoa Salad With Mediterranean Flavors

Ingredients

- One cup quinoa, one lemon,
- one teaspoon oregano,
- three-fourths teaspoon kosher salt,
- one-fourth teaspoon black pepper,
- one-fourth cup extra virgin olive oil, two bell peppers (orange, yellow, or red),
- half a cup of pitted, drained Kalamata olives,

- one English cucumber, and half a cup of crumbled feta cheese

Instructions

1. Prepare the quinoa. Under cold running water, give the quinoa a thorough rinse. Follow the directions on the box to cook.
2. Prepare the dressing. While the quinoa is cooking, combine the oregano, salt, pepper, and lemon juice and zest in a serving dish. Add the olive oil and whisk. To suit your tastes, taste the spice and adjust it.
3. Add some dressing to the quinoa. After cooking, add softened quinoa to the dressing bowl. Let the lemon dressing soak into the quinoa and stir to coat. Before you add the veggies, let it cool fully.
4. Chop the veggies and add them to the quinoa as you go as it cools. Cut the peppers into tiny pieces, trim and slice the scallions, then split the olives into smaller pieces with your knife. After cutting the cucumber in half, cut it into quarters. Stir in the basin. Add the feta last and serve. Although it is completely optional, you may add some flair by garnishing it with fresh oregano leaves.

Nutrition: per-serving

Calories:185.5 kcal

18.2g of carbohydrates and 5.7g of protein

10.6g of fat, 2 g of saturated fat.

1.6g of polyunsaturated fat, 6.2g of monounsaturated fat

5 mg of cholesterol

437.4 mg of sodium, Potassium: 257.8 mg

2.7g of fiber, 2.4g of sugar

1066.8 IU of vitamin A, 40.3 mg of vitamin C

27 mg of calcium, 1.4 milligrams of iron

Sweet Potato and Black Bean Salad

Ingredients

- One pound of sweet potatoes, peeled and sliced into cubes that are 3/4 inch
- Half a teaspoon of ground cumin, or more to taste, and three tablespoons of olive oil
- One-sixth teaspoon of optional red pepper flakes
- To taste, add ground black pepper and coarse salt.
- Two teaspoons of lime juice, freshly squeezed
- One 14.5-oz can of rinsed and drained black beans

- Half a cup of freshly chopped cilantro and one red onion, cut finely

Instructions

1. Turn the oven on to 450 degrees Fahrenheit (230 degrees Celsius).
2. Season sweet potatoes with cumin, pepper flakes, salt, and black pepper after drizzling them with 1 tablespoon olive oil on a rimmed baking sheet. Toss until coated evenly.
3. Place the lowest rack in the preheated oven and roast for 25 to 35 minutes, stirring halfway through, until the sweet potatoes are soft.
4. In a large bowl, whisk together the lime juice and the remaining 2 tablespoons of olive oil; add salt and black pepper to taste. Toss gently to coat the sweet potatoes, black beans, onion, and cilantro.

Nutrition: per-serving

4 Servings,

291 Calories

11g of total fat, 2g of saturated fat, and 462 milligrams of sodium

42g of total carbs, 11g of dietary fiber, and total sugars 8g

6g of protein, 11 mg of vitamin C

81 milligrams of calcium, 3 milligrams of iron

767 milligrams of potassium

Tuna And Avocado Salad

Ingredients

- One 5-ounce can of drained tuna, ideally packaged in olive oil
- Half a ripe avocado, cut approximately
- Half a cup of celery, chopped
- 1/4 cup of chopped red onions
- One tablespoon of extra virgin olive oil
- Two tablespoons of lemon juice
- Two tablespoons of freshly cut parsley or cilantro and one teaspoon of lemon zest
- Half a teaspoon of kosher salt
- Ground black pepper, fresh

Instructions

1. Mix: Fill a medium bowl with all of the ingredients. Using a fork, mix until all the ingredients are fully incorporated, breaking up the tuna bits and mashing the avocado.

2. Finish and serve: Top with toast or your preferred sandwich bread, and if needed, add more oil or salt and pepper.

Nutrition: per serving

2 servings

417 calories

31g of total fat, 5g of saturated fat, and 30 mg of cholesterol

631 mg of sodium, 19 grams of total carbohydrates.

12 grams of dietary fiber, Total Sugar 3g

21g of protein and 26 milligrams of vitamin C

Iron 2 mg and calcium 63 mg for

1101 milligrams of potassium

Mushrooms With Spinach Frittata

Ingredients

- Three-fourths of a pound of fresh mushrooms or other mushrooms ▢ Half a pound of spinach or comparable greensTwo chopped garlic cloves, three tablespoons of butter, salt, and black pepper, eight eggs, one-fourth cup of cream or milk, half a cup of shredded Gruyere cheese, and half a cup of grated Pecorino cheese

Instructions

1. For around 90 seconds, bring the spinach to a boil in salted water. After stopping the cooking by immersing in cold water, press the greens dry. Cut harshly. If necessary, this blanching may be completed a day in advance. You do this to keep the leaves' vibrant green color.
2. Heat the mushrooms in a 10-inch-wide cast iron pan over medium-high heat, stirring occasionally. They will eventually stop using water. Add the garlic and a pinch of salt when this occurs. After the majority of the water has evaporated, add the butter and heat until the mushrooms start to brown.
3. Whisk in the cheeses and chopped spinach after beating the eggs and cream.
4. Add the egg mixture and reduce the heat to medium-low. Make an effort to ensure that everything is spread evenly. Allow the frittata to gently cook for 10 to 15 minutes, or until the eggs are largely set.
5. To obtain some browning, you may finish the frittata under the broiler if you'd like. Before

slicing, remove and let it cool for five to ten minutes.

Nutrition: per serving

Calories:246 kcal

6 grams of carbohydrates.

17g of protein and 18g of fat , 9g of saturated fat

2 g of polyunsaturated fat, 5 g of monounsaturated fat.

1 g of trans fat, 255 mg of cholesterol

353 mg of sodium and 562 mg of potassium, 2 g of fiber.

1 g of sugar.

4192 IU of vitamin A

Iron: 9 mg, calcium: 310 mg, and vitamin C: 11 mg

Roasted Chicken and Vegetables Bowl

Ingredients

- Chicken Bite-sized portions of 10 oz/300 g skinless, boneless chicken thighs
- Two tablespoons of paprika
- One teaspoon of ground red pepper flakes

- Two tablespoons of dilly
- One garlic clove, salt, and pepper, minced
- One tablespoon of olive oil

Salad with Cabbage:

- Two cups of cabbage
- One cup of lettuce
- Tablespoon dill and one clove of garlic
- One teaspoon of salt, vinegar, and black pepper
- Chop two tablespoons of olives
- One teaspoon of olive oil
- Yogurt Yogurt with garlic sauce (1/2 cup)
- Two minced garlic cloves
- Three tablespoons of salt and dill
- Roasted veggies

Instructions

1. Make your veggies first using this recipe for spicy roasted vegetables. While the veggies are in the oven, you may do all of the next stages; just remember to check on them after 15 to 20 minutes.
2. Prepare the chicken. In a bowl or directly in the pan, combine the chicken and the remaining ingredients. Cover the pan and cook over medium-high heat for 3–4 minutes. Remove the

cover and continue to stir until the chicken is cooked, about 6–7 more minutes.

3. Put all of the salad's components in a bowl and thoroughly combine them. Before adding the other ingredients, I suggest rubbing the cabbage with a little salt and vinegar or lemon juice.

4. In a small bowl, combine the ingredients for the garlic sauce.

5. It's time to put your bowls together. Place the salad on the bottom, followed by the roasted veggies and chicken. Drizzle the sauce over everything and dig in!

Nutrition: per serving

2 Servings

Calories:445 kcal 24 g of fat.

6g of saturated fat, 0g of trans fat

17g of unsaturated fat, 186 mg of cholesterol

1118 mg of sodium, 21 g of carbohydrates.

7g of fiber, 9 g of sugar, 43 g of protein

Salmon and Avocado Salad

Ingredients

- Four cups of baby spinach, two chopped tomatoes, one chopped avocado, one chopped cucumber, peeled and sliced, one fourth cup of chopped red onion, two tablespoons of olive oil, two salmon filets, and salt and pepper to taste
- Dressing: 1 lemon vinegar recipe

Instructions

1. In a large pan, heat the olive oil over medium-high heat. Use salt and pepper to season the salmon filets. Cook for 4–5 minutes after adding the salmon filets, top side down.
2. Cook the salmon for a further two to three minutes after flipping it, or until it is largely opaque and yet has a hint of tenderness in the center.
3. Top with the cooked salmon after dividing the other salad ingredients into two bowls.
4. In a small dish, combine the dressing ingredients and pour over the food.

Nutrition: per-serving

Calories: 732 kcal,

21g of carbohydrates, 40g of protein, 56g of fat, 9g of saturated fat, 94 mg of cholesterol, 140 mg of sodium, 2180 mg of potassium, 11g of fiber, 8g of sugar, 6974 IU of vitamin A, 50 mg of vitamin C, 125 mg of calcium, and 4 mg of iron.

Cod With Green Beans And Tomatoes

Ingredients

4 8-ounce cod fillets◻1 pint cherry tomatoes◻12 ounces fresh green beans To taste, add salt and pepper. ◻One teaspoon of dried thyme, two tablespoons of olive oil, two tablespoons of lemon juice, and one-half teaspoon of garlic powder Delicious couscous to serve.◻For serving, chop the parsley.

Instructions

1. Turn the oven on to 400°F. Put parchment paper on a baking pan.
2. Using paper towels, pat dry the cod and arrange it in a single layer in the center of the sheet pan. Place the green beans on one side and the cherry tomatoes on the other. To taste, add salt and pepper to the veggies and cod.
3. Drizzle the fish with lemon juice and olive oil. Add garlic powder and thyme for seasoning. Apply the marinade to the cod using a brush or your hands, then brush any leftover marinade over the veggies.

4. Put the pan in the oven and bake for 12 to 15 minutes, or until the fish appears flaky and the tomatoes start to soften.
5. Spoon baking dish liquids over fish and serve with green beans and tomatoes over couscous or other grain.

Nutrition: per serving

Calories:299 kcal, 12g of carbohydrates, 43 g of protein, 9g of fat, 1g of saturated fat, 1g of polyunsaturated fat, and 5g of monounsaturated fat, 98 mg of cholesterol, 148 mg of sodium, 1388 mg of potassium, 3g of fiber, and 6g of sugar Iron: 3 mg, calcium: 86 mg, vitamin C: 43 mg, and vitamin A:

Seared Scallops With Broccoli And Carrots

5 servings

Ingredients

- 1 scallop, 1 broccoli, eight carrots, and one medium garlic. Abalone sauce with two cloves, 1.5 tablespoons water

Instructions:

1. Bring some water to a boil and add olive oil and sea salt. Set aside the scallops after blanching the broccoli and carrots.

2. Heat the oil in the pan, add the garlic, and cook until it starts to turn a light shade of brown. For a quick stir-fry, add the scallops, broccoli, and carrot.

3. Finally, add the abalone sauce and stir with a little amount of water. Serve and have fun!

Vegetables And Shrimp Stir-frying With Quinoa

Ingredients

- 1 cup cooked quinoa, 3 tablespoons extra virgin olive oil
- One cup of raw shrimp
- About 1 cup chopped broccoli, 1 red pepper,
- 1 cooked and chopped corn on the cob,
- 1 finely chopped onion, 2 carefully minced garlic cloves, 1 1/4 teaspoon paprika, 1 1/4 teaspoon ground cumin,
- 1 1/4 teaspoon powder ginger or freshly grated ginger, and 1 1/4 cup coconut milk
- To taste, add salt and pepper.

Instructions

1. After corn is cooked on the cob, put it aside.
2. Prepare the quinoa as directed on the box.

3. In the meanwhile, warm up three tablespoons of extra virgin olive oil in a big skillet.

4. Sauté the broccoli and red peppers for approximately three minutes, or until they are just beginning to soften.

5. Add the onions, garlic, shrimp, and corn. Next, add the ginger, cumin, and paprika. Just when the shrimp take on color, sauté them for two to three minutes.

6. Add coconut milk gradually. Mix the ingredients for one more minute.

7. Stir everything together after adding the cooked quinoa.

8. Add salt and pepper to taste.

Nutrition: per serving

Two servings

Calories:623 kcal, 71 g of carbohydrates, 15 g of protein, 33 g of fat, 9 g of saturated fat, 5 g of polyunsaturated fat, 17 g of monounsaturated fat, 1 g of trans fat, 19 mg of sodium, 838 mg of potassium, 9 g of fiber, 6 g of sugar, 1982 IU of vitamin A, 83 mg of vitamin C, 63 mg of calcium, and 6 mg of iron

Chicken with Zucchini Noodle Soup

Ingredients

- 1 pound of skinless, boneless chicken thighs or breast

- Two medium zucchinis.
- 4 cups of low-sodium chicken broth
- One tablespoon of olive oil
- One teaspoon of dried herbs, such as rosemary or thyme
- 1/4 teaspoon black pepper and 1/2 teaspoon salt
- 1/4 cup of optionally chopped fresh parsley
- 1/4 cup of optionally grated Parmesan cheese

Zucchini Noodles

Ingredients

- two medium zucchini
- Two teaspoons of olive oil
- To taste, add salt and pepper.

Instructions:

1. Heat the olive oil in a big saucepan over medium heat.
2. Add the chicken and simmer for 5 to 6 minutes, or until browned.
3. Season with salt, pepper, herbs, and chicken broth. Bring to a boil, then lower the heat and simmer until the chicken is cooked through, about 10 to 12 minutes.
4. Spiralize the zucchini into noodles while the chicken cooks.

5. Heat the olive oil in a different pan over medium heat. Cook the zucchini noodles for three to four minutes, or until they are just beginning to soften.
6. Remove the chicken from the saucepan and cut it into small pieces.
7. Stir the cooked zucchini noodles into the saucepan.
8. Put the chicken back in the saucepan and boil it for two to three more minutes.
9. If necessary, taste and adjust the seasoning.
10. If wanted, top with Parmesan cheese and parsley and serve hot.

Nutrition: per serving
Calories: 250 kcal
35 g of protein, 10g of fat
25 g of carbohydrates, 5 g of fiber.
5 g of sugar, 500 mg of sodium

Lemon Herb Chicken with Roasted Sweet Potato Marinade

Ingredients
- One pound of chicken breasts
- Two teaspoons of freshly cut, finely chopped rosemary
- Two teaspoons of freshly chopped thyme
- One tablespoon of lemon juice

- To taste, add one teaspoon of sea salt and black pepper.
- One sliced onion
- One and a half pounds of diced sweet potatoes, one tablespoon of olive oil, and salt and pepper to taste
- One pound of finely chopped broccoli
- One sliced red bell pepper
- One lemon, cut thinly

Instructions

1. Set the oven's temperature to 450 degrees F.
2. Add the chicken to a bowl after chopping it into big chunks.
3. Toss the chicken in a bowl with chopped herbs, lemon juice, sea salt, and black pepper. Stir well, then place in the refrigerator to marinate while the veggies are being prepared.
4. Spread 1 tablespoon of olive oil on a sheet pan to coat it.
5. Season with sea salt and pepper to taste, add the chopped onion and big sweet potato cubes to the pan, and bake for 15 minutes.
6. After fifteen minutes, remove the pan and surround it with the chicken. Return to the oven for ten more minutes.

7. Remove the pan again and add the lemon slices, red bell pepper, and broccoli. Return to the oven and bake for ten minutes.
8. While everything is still hot, serve straight from the oven. All the wonderful tastes are absorbed by the onions in the bottom of the pan!

Nutrition: per serving

Calories: 381 kcal, 50g of carbohydrates, 31g of protein, 7g of fat, 1g of saturated fat, 73 mg of cholesterol, 848 mg of sodium, 1522 mg of potassium, 11g of fiber, 12g of sugar, 26001 IU of vitamin A, 169 mg of vitamin C, 150 mg of calcium, and 4 mg of iron.

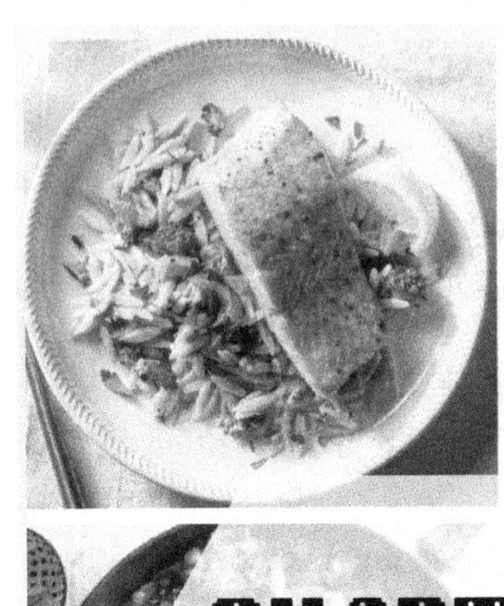
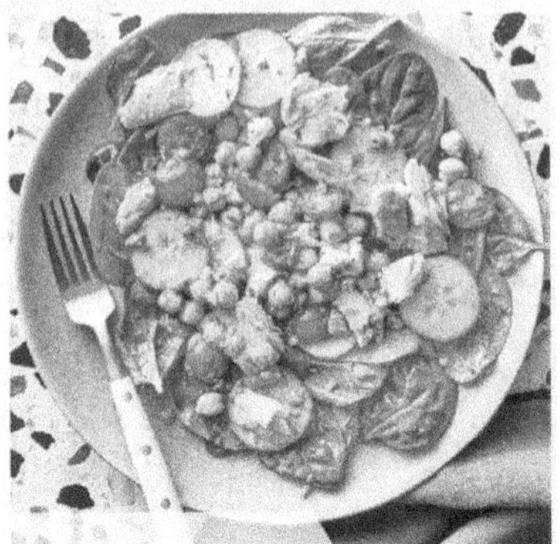

CHAPTER SIX

REFRESHING ANTI INFLAMMATORY DINNER RECIPES

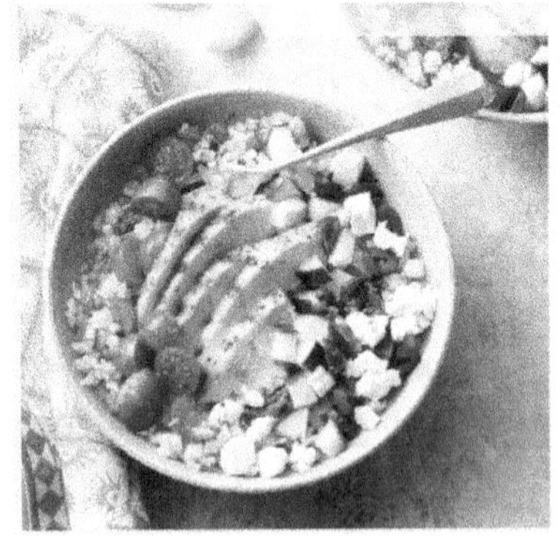
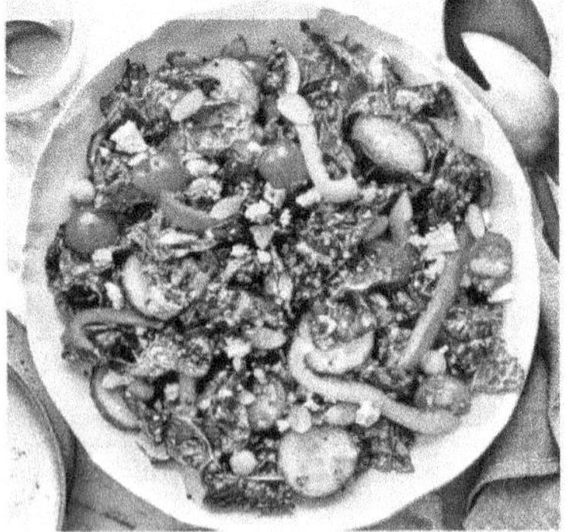

CHAPTER 6

DINNER RECIPES

Zucchini Noodles Pad Thai

Ingredients

- Three huge zucchinis.
- Half a cup of chicken stock
- 2 ½ teaspoons of pasted tamarind
- Two teaspoons of soy sauce with reduced sodium
- Two teaspoons of oyster sauce
- One and a half teaspoons of Asian chili sauce
- One tablespoon of Worcestershire sauce
- One tablespoon of freshly squeezed lime juice
- One spoonful of white sugar
- A pair of teaspoons of sesame oil
- One tablespoon of finely chopped garlic
- 12 ounces of chicken breasts, cut into 1-inch cubes, without the skin or bones
- Eight ounces of diced and peeled shrimp
- Two beaten eggs and two tablespoons of water, or as necessary (optional)
- Three cups of bean sprouts, separated
- Cut six green onions into 1-inch slices.

- Two teaspoons of dry-roasted peanuts, chopped and unsalted
- Half a cup of freshly chopped basil

Instructions

1. Spiralize the zucchini to make noodles.
2. In a small bowl, whisk together the chicken stock, tamarind paste, soy sauce, oyster sauce, Worcestershire sauce, chile pepper sauce, lime juice, and sugar to create a smooth sauce.
3. In a large skillet or wok, heat the sesame oil over high heat. Stir in garlic for ten seconds or until fragrant. Add the chicken and shrimp, and cook and stir for 5 to 7 minutes, or until the chicken is no longer pink in the middle and the juices run clear.
4. To create a space in the middle of the wok, push the shrimp and chicken to the sides. Scramble the eggs for two to three minutes until they are hard. Add the sauce and zucchini noodles; simmer for approximately three minutes, stirring occasionally and adding water as necessary. Cook and stir for 1 to 2 minutes after adding 2 cups of bean sprouts and green onions.
5. Take off the heat and top the noodles with peanuts. Garnish with fresh basil and the remaining cup of bean sprouts.

Nutrition: Per-serving

Four servings

Calories: 370 kcal, 15g of total fat, 3g of saturated fat, and 222 mg of cholesterol

671 mg of sodium

28g of total carbohydrates, 5g of dietary fiber, 13g of total sugars, and 36g of protein

56 mg of vitamin C

Iron 5 mg, potassium 1141 mg, and calcium 121 mg

Baked Salmon With Cauliflower And Broccoli

Ingredients

- One tablespoon of olive oil
- One lemon and its juice
- 1/2 teaspoon of powdered garlic
- Half a teaspoon of red pepper flakes
- Two cups of florcts of broccoli
- Two cups of cauliflower
- Four 4-ounce salmon filets
- To taste, add salt and pepper.

Instructions

1. Set the oven's temperature to 400°F.
2. On a sheet pan, arrange the cauliflower florets and broccoli. Add lemon juice, red pepper flakes, garlic, olive oil, salt, and pepper for seasoning. For 8 to 10 minutes, bake.
3. After taking the sheet pan out of the oven, place the salmon filets in the middle of it. Add salt, pepper, lemon juice, red pepper flakes, olive oil, and garlic to the fish. The salmon should be cooked to your taste after another 10 to 15 minutes in the oven.
4. Serve right away or keep in the fridge for up to three days.

Nutrition: per-serving

242 calories (kcal)

12g of total fat, 2g of saturated fat, and 0g of trans fat

72g of cholesterol and 228 mg of sodium

6g of total carbohydrates and 2g of dietary fiber

Added Sugars 2g, Total Sugars 28g, of protein (0g)

0 mg of vitamin D

Iron 2 mg, calcium 46 mg, 933 milligrams of potassium

Grilled Shrimp And Veggie Skewers

Ingredients

Supplies for the Shrimp (enough to create four skewers)

- One pound of big, peeled, and deveined shrimp
- Half a cup of plain, fat-free Greek yogurt
- One-fourth cup lemon juice
- Half a teaspoon each of oregano and dill
- Half a teaspoon of kosher salt
- Two cloves of garlic
- For the vegetables (each skewer yields eight)
- One pint of cherry tomatoes
- One bunch of asparagus
- One red onion
- Red wine vinegar (one tablespoon)
- One teaspoon of olive oil
- Half a teaspoon of kosher salt
- 1/4 teaspoon dried dill
- 1/4 teaspoon dried oregano
- Two garlic cloves

Instructions

1. To make the marinade, combine all the ingredients (except the shrimp) and whisk to combine.
2. Add the marinade to the shrimp. To marinate, cover and refrigerate for at least 4 hours.
3. Put the shrimp on metal or wooden skewers. To soften your skewers while using an outside barbecue, immerse them in water. This is not essential if you are using a grill pan.
4. Cook over medium-high heat in a grill pan or on a grill, turning once until cooked through.
5. Regarding the vegetables
6. Clean the veggies. Cut the asparagus's end off.
7. Cut the onion into large enough pieces to fit on a skewer. Cut the asparagus into pieces that are 1.5 to 2".
8. To make the vinaigrette, combine all the ingredients (excluding the veggies) in a small bowl.
9. Alternately skewer the veggies in a pattern on metal or wooden skewers. To soften your skewers while using an outside barbecue, immerse them in water. This is not essential if you are using a grill pan.
10. Transfer the skewers to a platter and cover them with the vinaigrette.
11. Until you're ready to prepare the veggies, let them sit.

12. If using a grill pan, cook the veggies for around ten minutes, covering with a lid and turning often.

13. Before serving, drizzle the grilled skewers with the leftover vinaigrette from the dish.

Nutrition: per serving

Four servings

Calories: 201 kcal, 15 g of carbohydrates , 30 g of protein, 3 g of fat ,1 g of saturated fat, 1 g of trans fat, 287 mg of cholesterol, 1489 mg of sodium, 685 mg of potassium, 4 g of fiber, 7 g of sugar, 1440 IU of vitamin A, 47 mg of vitamin C, 251 mg of calcium, 6 mg of iron.

Spaghetti Squash With Meat Sauce

Ingredients

- One small spaghetti squash (two pounds) , one tablespoon of avocado oil, one pound of lean ground beef, and one tiny diced onion (4 ounces).
- Two cups of marinara sauce, two teaspoons of minced parsley, two tablespoons of grated Parmesan, and one-sixth teaspoon of Diamond Crystal kosher salt and black pepper

Instructions

Get the squash ready:

1. Using a sharp knife, make a few punctures in the spaghetti squash. After 5 minutes, flip it and microwave for 5 more minutes until tender. To complete cooking, let it stand for five minutes.
2. Cut the spaghetti squash in half lengthwise with a sharp knife. Let it cool for five minutes, or until it becomes manageable. Using a fork, rake the flesh strands out onto a serving dish after scooping away the pulp and seeds from the center. Put aside.

Prepare the sauce:

1. In a large, deep saucepan, heat the oil over medium-high heat for about three minutes. Add salt, pepper, onions, and meat. Sauté the beef for around five minutes, breaking it up as you cook, until it is no longer raw.
2. Add the marinara sauce and stir. Reduce the heat to medium-low and simmer, covered, stirring periodically, for 20 minutes after bringing to a boil.

Complete the dish:

1. Serve the beef sauce by ladling it over the squash noodles and garnishing it with Parmesan and parsley.

Nutrition: per-serving

Four Servings

Calories: 407 kcal, 14 g of carbohydrates, 24 g of protein, 28 g of fat, 9 g of saturated fat, 624 mg of sodium, 3 g of fiber, 7 g of sugar.

Lentil and Vegetable Stew

Ingredients

- 2 tablespoons of olive oil.
- Four garlic cloves and one yellow onion
- Four carrots (about half a pound)
- Four celery stalks
- Two pounds of potatoes
- One cup of brown lentils
- Dried rosemary, 1 teaspoon.
- Half a teaspoon of dried thyme
- Two tablespoons Dijon mustard
- 1.5 tablespoons of soy sauce
- One tablespoon of brown sugar
- One cup of frozen peas and six glasses of vegetable broth

Instructions

1. Chop the garlic and dice the onion. In a large soup pot, add the olive oil, onion, and garlic. Over medium heat, start to sauté them.

2. Add the celery to the saucepan and continue to sauté it after chopping the onion and garlic. Peel and cut the carrots into half rounds while the celery, onion, and garlic are sautéing. Continue to sauté the carrots after adding them to the saucepan.

3. Peel the potatoes and cube them into 3/4 to 1-inch pieces while the carrots, celery, onion, and garlic are sautéing. Add the lentils, Dijon, thyme, rosemary, brown sugar, soy sauce, and vegetable broth to the saucepan with the diced potatoes.

4. Stir the ingredients together for a few seconds, then cover the pot, increase the heat to high, and bring the stew to a boil. After it comes to a boil, reduce the heat to low and simmer it for half an hour, stirring now and again.

5. When the potatoes are extremely tender, at the end of the simmering period, start mashing them a little while stirring. The stew will become thicker as a result.

6. Lastly, toss in the frozen peas and let them warm through after 30 minutes. If necessary, add salt to the stew, Enjoy it!

Nutrition: per-serving

249.2 kcal

45.91 g of carbohydrates.

9.88g of protein, 3.99g of fat

964.61 mg of sodium, 7.86g of fiber

Chickpea and Vegetable Curry

Ingredients

- Twice as much vegetable oil
- One little onion, diced; two smashed garlic cloves
- Three tablespoons of curry powder
- 225g of peeled and sliced carrots
- 225 grams of quartered mushrooms.
- One little cauliflower head, divided into two
- Two tablespoons of tomato purée
- 225g of chopped tomatoes in a can
- 600 milliliters of vegetable stock
- 410g can of rinsed and drained chickpeas (or any other bean of your choosing)
- One hundred grams of frozen peas

- 200g of basmati rice (or 50g per person), cooked according to the package's directions

Instructions

1. In a big saucepan, heat the oil and cook the onion gently for two minutes. (While the oil is heated, drop a slice of onion into it.) The oil is ready when the onion begins to sizzle.
2. After adding the curry powder and garlic and stirring to coat the onions and garlic well, let the mixture simmer for two minutes. If you're not sure how hot you want your curry, start with less curry powder and add more as you want.
3. Add the cauliflower, carrots, and mushrooms and continue to cook gently for three more minutes.
4. Stir in the chickpeas after adding the stock, canned tomatoes, and tomato purée. Bring to a boil.
5. After ten minutes of gentle simmering, add the peas and mix. The moment to begin making your rice is now!
6. Serve over rice after another 10 minutes of cooking and seasoning to taste.

Roasted Turkey With Brussel Sprouts And Butternut Squash

Ingredients

- Extra Lean Ground Turkey, 1 pound
- Four to six pieces of nitrate-free bacon
- One teaspoon of cinnamon
- Two tablespoons of poultry seasoning, sometimes known as "Thanksgiving spice blend,"
- One tablespoon of avocado oil
- One cup of chopped red onion
- A tablespoon of minced garlic
- Two cups of clipped and halved Brussels sprouts
- Two cups of diced and peeled butternut squash
- Two medium apples (diced and cored)
- Half a teaspoon of sea salt

Instructions

1. A big skillet should be heated to medium heat. Add the poultry seasoning, cinnamon, and ground turkey. Cook, breaking it into small pieces as it cooks, until well browned, 5 to 7 minutes. After removing the fat, move it to a dish and put it away.
2. Cook your bacon strips in a different, smaller pan for around five to seven minutes.
3. Heat the oil in the same skillet over medium heat. Sauté the garlic and onion until they become transparent. Add the apples, butternut squash, and Brussels sprouts after that. Cover and boil, stirring occasionally, until all vegetables are tender, approximately 10 minutes.

4. Return the ground turkey to the skillet and mix everything together. Mix everything together after adding the bacon and bacon fat. Enjoy after dividing into portions!

Nutrition: per-serving

Calories: 680 kcal

59 g of protein, 43 g of fat.

12g of saturated fat, 32 g of carbohydrates.

10g of fiber, 15g of sugar

Grilled Swordfish with Mango Salad

Ingredients

- 2 mangos, 1 lemon, 2 tablespoons vegetable oil, 1 teaspoon of cumin powder, 1 teaspoon salt, 1 jalapeño, 4 green onions, 1/2 red onion, 1/2 red bell pepper, 1/2 yellow bell pepper, and 1/4 cup fresh cilantro

Instructions

1. Salsa with mangoes, Lemon juice, oil, kosher salt, freshly cracked black pepper, and a sprinkle

of cumin powder should all be whisked together in a dish.

2. To coat and marinate, add the mango chunks and mix.
3. Add the chopped bell peppers, cilantro, green onions, and half of a red onion to the mango dish.
4. Slice off the jalapeño pepper's stem while wearing latex or rubber gloves. Then, remove the seed and white membrane and dispose of them. Add the finely chopped pepper to the bowl.
5. Toss to coat, then refrigerate for 30 minutes to marinate.

Preparing the Swordfish

1. Turn the grill on to 500°F. Season your swordfish with salt and pepper before grilling.
2. After cleaning the grill, place swordfish on it and reduce the heat to 400°F. For a soft, cooked-through swordfish, I want mine to have grill marks, and two to three minutes on each side should be plenty. If you overcook it, it will become dry. The fish should be cooked uniformly and moistly.

Nutrition: per-serving

Calories: 89 kcal, 12 g of carbohydrates, 1 g of protein, 4 g of fat, 3 g of saturated fat, 391 mg of sodium, 194 mg of potassium, 2 g of fiber, 9 g of sugar, 1075 IU of vitamin A, 65.6 mg of vitamin C, 19 mg of calcium, and 0.4 mg of iron

Lobster Tail with Lemon and Asparagus

Ingredients

- 400 g asparagus spears, 200 g snow peas, and three green lobster tails
- 30 grams of butter
- Four chopped green onions
- One-third cup of lemon juice and two tablespoons of lemon zest
- One-third cup of pine nuts

Instructions

1. Using scissors, cut the lobster tails down either side of the bottom.
2. Slice the lobster thickly after removing the meat from the shells.
3. Put the snow peas on top and tail them.
4. Slice off the asparagus's woody end.
5. Bring the asparagus to a boil, steam, or microwave until it is just beginning to soften, then add the snow peas and continue cooking for another minute. After draining, rinse with cold water until it's no longer heated.

6. Add the green onions, lemon rind, and juice to a skillet with heated butter.

7. Add the snow peas, asparagus, and pine nuts after the lobster has been stir-fried until it is just soft. Stir until well heated.

Stir-fried Chicken With Brown rice And Broccoli

Two servings

Ingredients

- 200g of chopped and halved broccoli florets
- One local organic chicken breast, chopped; fifteen grams of ginger, shredded
- Two cloves of garlic, chopped into shreds
- One sliced red onion
- One cube of roasted red pepper
- Two teaspoons of extra-vigor olive oil
- One teaspoon of mild chili powder
- One tablespoon of tamari sauce
- Brown rice with 1 tablespoon of honey.

Instructions

1. Place the broccoli in a medium pan that is ready to be heated and set the kettle to a boil. After

adding the water, let the broccoli boil for two minutes.

2. In a non-stick pan, heat the olive oil and stir-fry the onion, ginger, and garlic for two minutes. Then, add the mild chili powder and stir just a little.
3. Stir-fry the chicken for another two minutes. Save the water after draining the broccoli.
4. Add the broccoli to the pan along with the red pepper, honey, soy, and four tablespoons of broccoli water. Cook until the broccoli is well cooked.
5. In the meantime, prepare the rice and serve it with the stir-fry.

Portobello Buns And Grilled Turkey Burger

Ingredients

- 1 tablespoon of olive oil and 1 pound of ground turkey breast
- Six peeled garlic cloves
- One red onion, cut thinly
- Thinly cut six ounces of portabella, eight ounces of button, or six ounces of cremini mushrooms.
- One tablespoon of balsamic acid
- One tablespoon of Dijon mustard

- One teaspoon of crushed dried rosemary
- One teaspoon tamari, or low-sodium soy sauce,
- One-half teaspoon of salt, to taste
- One-half teaspoon of pepper, to taste
- Three teaspoons of shredded blue cheese
- Four ciabatta bread, four kaiser rolls, or four sourdough French rolls, with salad greens as an optional garnish

Instructions

1. Remove the grates from the grill and prepare it for direct-heat cooking. Instead of using the grill, we utilized a stovetop grill pan.
2. Heat the oil in a nonstick skillet over medium high heat.
3. Cook the garlic cloves until they are just beginning to brown.
4. To ensure uniform browning, turn the cloves as necessary.
5. To cool, transfer to a cutting board.
6. Cook the tamari sauce and onion slices in the remaining oil in a pan until they are soft.
7. Add the mushrooms and simmer until they are soft.
8. Stir in the balsamic vinegar for approximately 30 seconds, or until it almost evaporates.
9. Take off the heat and let it cool a little while you make the burgers.

10. Chop and dd the garlic, turkey, mustard, rosemary, salt, and pepper to a medium-sized bowl.
11. Form into four 4-inch-diameter burgers.
12. Apply a little cooking spray on the grill pan to prepare it, or spray the great and lay it over hot embers.
13. Burgers should be grilled for 5 minutes on each side, or until the center is no longer pink (165°F).
14. On sourdough French, Kaiser, or ciabatta buns, arrange the burgers and mixed greens.
15. Top the burgers with a spoonful of the bleu cheese after stirring it into the mushroom mixture.
16. Enjoy it with sliced tomatoes and fries!

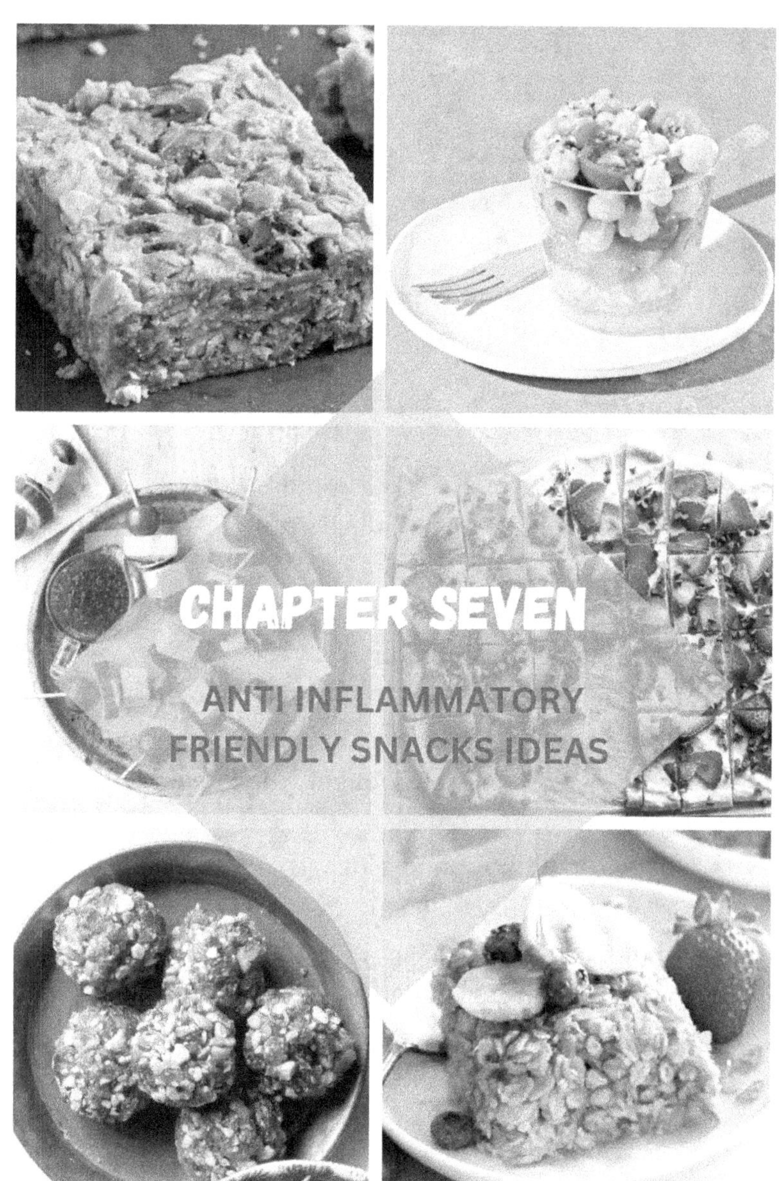

CHAPTER SEVEN

ANTI INFLAMMATORY FRIENDLY SNACKS IDEAS

CHAPTER 7

SNACKS AND SIDES

Coconut Yogurt Parfait With Berries And Granola

Ingredients

- Cut two cups of strawberries into slices.
- One and a half cups of blueberries
- Half a cup of coconut shreds
- Twenty ounces of four separate dairy-free vanilla, strawberry, blueberry, or strawberry yogurts (you may, of course, use normal yogurt if you like)
- Two cups of granola may be made using the recipe below or store-bought, for a total of four cups.
- Regarding the almond-blueberry granola
- Two cups of dry oatmeal
- Half a cup of blueberries, dried
- Half a cup of raw almonds, sliced
- Half a cup of brown rice syrup
- One tablespoon of coconut oil
- Two tablespoons of whole flaxseed

- One teaspoon of cinnamon, 1/2 tablespoon vanilla extract 1/4 TSP salt

Instructions

1. Preheat the oven to 325 degrees before beginning to create the homemade granola (or go on to step 8). Apply cooking spray on a baking sheet.
2. Heat the brown rice syrup, coconut oil, salt, cinnamon, and vanilla essence in a small saucepan over medium-low heat. Until the mixture begins to boil, stir frequently. Take off the heat.
3. In a medium bowl, mix together the oats, almonds, blueberries, and flaxseeds, stirring to combine. After adding the wet mixture, use a wooden spoon to mix it evenly.
4. Evenly distribute the granola mixture over the pan.
5. Bake for eight minutes. Flip the granola over with a spatula and stir. The granola should be gently toasted after 8 more minutes of cooking in the oven.
6. To cool for a few minutes, place the baking sheet on a wire rack. When the granola has cooled a little, break it off the baking sheet in clusters using the back of a spatula.

7. For the parfaits, measure out two cups of the granola. For later use, move the remainder to a dish or container.

8. In four glasses, start stacking your parfaits: First, fill each cup with half of the yogurt. Next, evenly distribute 1 cup of granola (1/4 cup in each cup) over the yogurt. Next, fill each cup with half a cup of strawberries. Cover with a layer of the remaining yogurt. The remaining granola (1/4 cup each), shredded coconut (2 TBSP each), and blueberries (1/3 cup each) should then be added.

9. Either serve right away or keep in the refrigerator until you're ready to serve.

Nutrition: per-serving

Calories: 510 kcal

85 g of carbohydrates, 12g of protein and 15g of fat

6g of saturated fat, 10g of fiber, 40g of sugar.

Apple Slices with Almond Butter

Ingredients

- Apples, 1 tablespoon of almond butter (available at the grocery store)

Instructions

1. Slice and core the apple.
2. Top apple slices with almond butter and dig in!

Nutrition: Per-serving

426 kJ of energy

2.3g of protein, 8.1g of carbohydrates

6.1g of total fat and 0.8g of saturated fat

3.1g of fiber, 45.8 mg of sodium

Turmeric Roasted Chickpeas:

Ingredients

- 400 grams of canned chicken
- Red paprika and three tablespoons of olive oil
- Half a teaspoon of turmeric, cayenne pepper, salt, ginger, thyme, and oregano

Instructions

1. Turn the oven on to 200°C (390°F).
2. After draining, rinse and pat dry the chickpeas. You may remove any skin that falls off, but it's not required. Dry your chickpeas thoroughly with paper towels.

3. Add your spices to a bowl with olive oil. A sprinkle of cayenne pepper, a pinch of salt, a pinch of ginger, thyme, oregano, half a teaspoon of turmeric, and one teaspoon of red paprika. Mix thoroughly.
4. Toss to mix the dry chickpeas with the olive oil coating.
5. After coating the chickpeas, place them on a baking pan lined with aluminum foil or baking paper. Bake them for approximately half an hour, or until they are golden brown. Take out of the oven and let cool. The chickpeas will get crispy as they cool. Serve as a snack or as a garnish for salads or soups.

Nutrition: per serving

Six servings

Calories:156 kcal

9 g of fat, 1g of saturated fat, 0g of trans fat, 7g of unsaturated fat, 0 mg of cholesterol, 262 milligrams of sodium, 16g of carbohydrate, 5 g of fiber, 3 g of sugar, 5 g of protein.

Lemon Tahini Dip with Kale Chips

Ingredients

- One bunch of kale chopped into small pieces
- Half a cup of creamy tahini
- Two tablespoons of lemon juice
- One tablespoon of spice for steak
- Red pepper flakes, ¼ teaspoon
- Four tablespoons of olive or avocado oil

Instructions

1. Set the oven temperature to 350 degrees. In a small bowl, combine all the ingredients except the kale.
2. Place the kale in a big bowl after tearing or chopping it to the appropriate size. Pour in some oil. The stems may be left in place. Evenly coat the kale with half of the tahini mixture by massaging it in.
3. Use silicone mats or foil to line the baking pan. Lay the kale flat on the baking sheet that has been prepared, taking care not to pack it too full. Working in two batches could be required of you. Bake until crispy, 10 to 12 minutes.
4. Take it out of the oven and let it cool. Serve the leftover tahini sauce on the side.

Nutrition: per-serving

218 kcal, 4g of carbohydrates, 3g of protein, 22g of fat, 3g of saturated fat, 5g of polyunsaturated fat, 13g of

monounsaturated fat, 8 mg of sodium, 87 mg of potassium, 1g of fiber, 0.2 g of sugar99 IU of vitamin A, 4 mg of vitamin C, 33 mg of calcium, and 1 mg of iron

Baked Sweet Potato Chips

Ingredients

- Two 150-gram organic sweet potatoes
- Two tablespoons of olive oil
- 1/4 teaspoon sea salt, if desired

Instructions

1. Place the oven rack in the middle of the oven and preheat it to 250 degrees Fahrenheit (121 degrees Celsius).

2. After giving your sweet potatoes a thorough rinse and drying, cut them into slices that are as thin as possible (about 1/8 to 1/16 inches thick). Make advantage of your mandolin if you have one. If not, thin them evenly with a very sharp knife. Be aware that partially thick chips will not crisp up completely. Not "chip" crispiness, but still excellent.

3. Sprinkle the slices with salt after tossing them in a little olive oil to gently coat them. Arrange in a single layer on a baking sheet coated with parchment paper, and bake for about one hour thirty to one hour forty-five minutes, turning the chips once halfway through to guarantee even

cooking. For more consistent cooking, I also turned mine, which is optional but advised. Note: Cooking time will be affected by slice thickness. Make sure they aren't burning by checking them every ten minutes or so throughout the second hour of cooking.

4. When golden brown and crisp, remove. Before tasting, remove any that feel a bit sensitive in the center and let them sit for fifteen minutes or so to crisp up. Serve right away.

Nutrition : per-serving
Two servings
Calories:248 kcal
30.2 g of carbohydrates and 2.4 g of protein
13.6 g of fat, 1.9 g of saturated fat
1.44 g of polyunsaturated fat
9.85 g of monounsaturated fat
0 g of trans fat, 0 mg of cholesterol.
83 mg of sodium, 506 milligrams of potassium
4.5 g of fiber, 6.3 g of sugar
21281 IU of vitamin A
3.6 milligrams of vitamin C
45.14 mg of calcium, 0.99 mg of iron

Slices Of Bell Pepper With Hummus Dip With Carrots

Ingredients

- 3/4 cup of hummus
- Half a cup of baby carrots, whole
- Half a medium pepper or two sliced red bell peppers

Instructions

1. If you want to take hummus as a snack, put it in a bowl or mason jar.
2. Cut bell peppers and carrots into long, thin strips.
3. Dip and savor!

Nutrition: per serving

471 calories, 290 calories from fat, 38 calories from saturated fat, 32 grams of total fat, 4.2 grams of saturated fat, 0.0 grams of trans fat, 14.1 grams of polyunsaturated fat, 11.9 grams of monounsaturated fat, 0 cholesterol, 868 mg of sodium, 810 mg of potassium, 37 grams of dietary fiber, 12.6 grams of sugar, S5.4 grams, and 14.7 grams of protein.

Garlic and Herb Roasted Carrots.

Ingredients

- ½ teaspoon garlic powder, ½ teaspoon dried oregano, ½ teaspoon dried basil, ½ teaspoon dried parsley, ½ teaspoon dried thyme, ½ teaspoon salt (or to taste), ¼ teaspoon pepper (or to taste), 1 pound of freshly washed carrots, and two tablespoons olive oil

Instructions

1. Turn the oven on to 425°F. Apply cooking spray to a baking sheet to lightly coat it.

2. Combine the garlic, oregano, basil, parsley, thyme, salt, and pepper in a small bowl. Drizzle the carrots with 2 tablespoons of olive oil and the garlic-herb combination. Combine all the ingredients, adding the garlic and herb combination to each carrot.

3. On the baking sheet, arrange the carrots in a single layer. Bake for 25 to 30 minutes, or until they are fork tender.

Nutrition: per-serving

Calories: 111 kcal, 11 grams of carbohydrates.

1 g of protein, 7 g of fat.

1g of saturated fat

370 mg of sodium and 363 milligrams of potassium
3 g of fiber, 5g of sugar, 18944 IU of vitamin A
7 mg of vitamin C, 37 mg of calcium
Iron: 1 mg (6% LK)

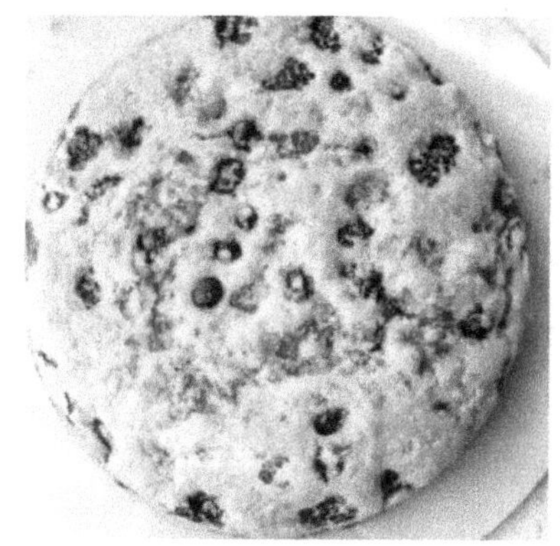
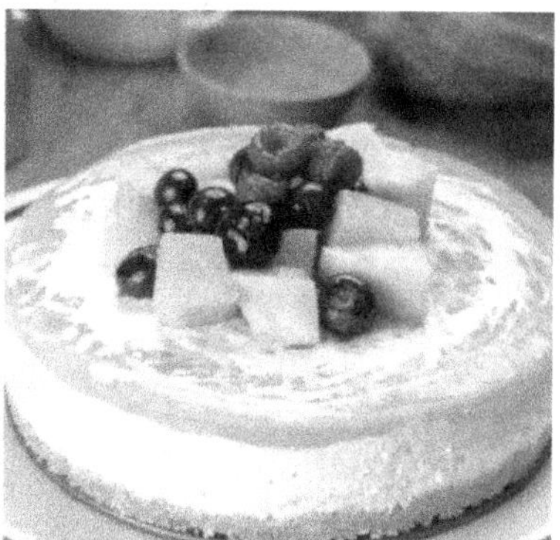

CHAPTER EIGHT

ANTI INFLAMMATORY DESSERT RECIPES

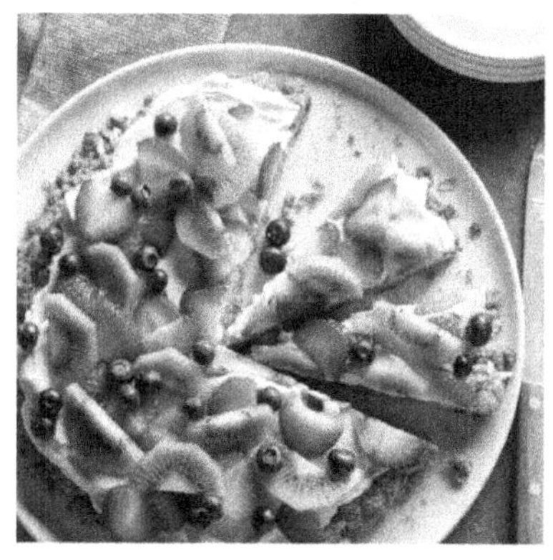
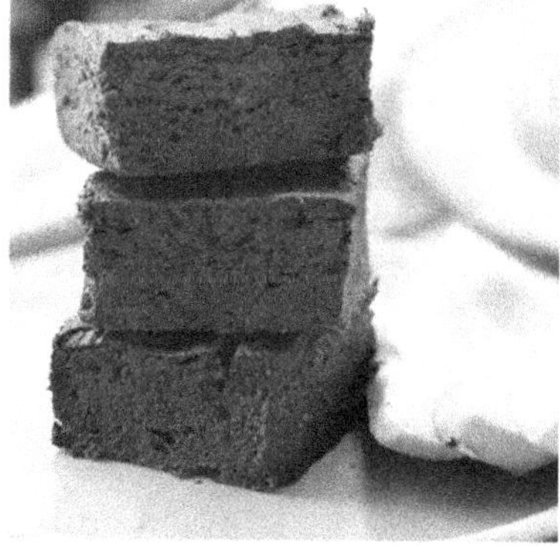

CHAPTER 8

DESSERT

Blueberry Oatmeal Bars

Ingredients

- One cup of whole oatmeal
- One cup of oat flour
- Half a cup of brown sugar
- Half a teaspoon each of baking soda and salt
- Half a cup almond milk
- Two eggs
- Half a cup of melted butter
- One teaspoon of vanilla extract
- One cup of fresh blueberries
- 1/4 cup of walnuts, chopped
- ⅓ cup optionally shredded coconut

Instructions

1. Turn the oven on to 175 degrees Celsius (350 degrees Fahrenheit). Grease a pan that is 8 inches square.
2. In a bowl, mix together whole oats, oat flour, brown sugar, baking soda, and salt. Add the eggs, butter, almond milk, and vanilla and stir until

completely blended. Stir in walnuts and blueberries. Cover the prepared pan with the mixture and sprinkle the coconut shreds on top.

3. Bake for approximately 35 minutes in a preheated oven, or until the coconut is caramelized and the edges are golden. After 10 minutes of cooling in the pan, cut into 16 squares.

Nutrition: per-serving

For eight servings

Calories: 324 kcal.

16g of total fat, 6g of saturated fat, and 62 mg of cholesterol, 305 milligrams of sodium, Dietary Fiber 4g, Total Sugars 41g, Total Carbohydrates 18g, 8 g of Protein, 2 mg of Vitamin C, Iron 2 mg and calcium 59 mg, 237 milligrams of potassium

Chocolate Avocado Mousse

Ingredients

- Half a pitted, peeled, and diced avocado
- Five tablespoons of cacao powder or unsweetened cocoa powder

- ¾ cup full-fat coconut milk (use just the thick, creamy portion after refrigerating the can for at least 4 hours).
- Two and a half tablespoons of pure maple syrup, date paste, or agave nectar
- One-sixth teaspoon sea salt, and one-sixth teaspoon optional vanilla essence.

Instructions

1. Put all the ingredients in a food processor or blender set to high speed.
2. After approximately 20 seconds of blending, stop and scrape down the sides of the jug.
3. Continue until the mousse is lump-free and silky.
4. Transfer into two serving dishes and garnish with cacao powder, grated chocolate, whipped cream, or fresh berries.

Nutrition: Per-serving

Calories: 353 kcal

31.3g of carbohydrates, 5g of protein, 28.2g of fat, 21.1g of saturated fat, 78 mg of sodium, 748 mg of potassium, 13g of fiber, 18.3g of sugar, 49 mg of calcium, and 4 mg of iron

Berry Chia Seed Pudding

Ingredients

- 1 cup of your preferred berries.
- One cup of plant-based milk
- One teaspoon of maple syrup
- Three tablespoons of chia seeds
- One cup of vegan yogurt

Instructions

In a blender, combine together the berries, maple syrup, and plant-based milk until smooth.

Pour the chia seeds into a dish with the berry milk. Give it at least two hours to set in the refrigerator. Serve as a tasty addition to porridge or with vegan yogurt. Keep in the refrigerator for up to three days.

Nutrition: per-serving

Two servings

Calories: 244.7 kcal, 29.7 g of carbohydrates, 9.6 g of protein, 10.1 g of fat, 1.1 g of saturated fat, 5.8 g of polyunsaturated fat, 0.9 g of monounsaturated fat, 0.03 g of trans fat, 77.3 mg of sodium, 268.4 mg of potassium, 8.2 g of fiber, 14.4 g of sugar, 491.3 IU of vitamin A,

24.7 mg of vitamin C, 435.5 mg of calcium, and 2 mg of iron.

Sweet Potato Brownies

Ingredients

- One cup of mashed cooked sweet potatoes, half a cup of almond butter (which may be substituted for any kind of nut or seed butter), three tablespoons of maple syrup, 1/4 cup of cocoa powder, and half a cup of chocolate chips Not required.

Instructions

1. Grease a loaf pan and put aside after preheating the oven to 180°C (350°F).
2. Put all the ingredients in a high-speed blender or food processor and pulse until the batter is smooth.
3. After the pan has been oiled, pour the mixture into it and bake it for about 20 minutes, or until it is well cooked. Take it out of the oven and let it cool fully. Frost if you like, then cut into slices.

Nutrition: per-serving

Calories: 185 kcal

12 g of carbohydrates, 5 g of protein.

19 g of fat, 3 milligrams of potassium

6g of fiber, 150 IU of vitamin A

2.5 milligrams of vitamin C, 30 mg of calcium

0.5 milligrams of iron, 6g of net carbs

Frozen Yogurt Bark With Berries And Nuts

Ingredient

- Two cups of vanilla yogurt, one-half cup of cut strawberries, and one-half cup of pistachios or any other granola or nuts

Instructions

1. Put parchment paper on a baking pan.
2. Using an offset spatula, spread the yogurt on the sheet pan.
3. Evenly distribute the cut pistachios and strawberries over it.
4. Freeze for at least three hours or overnight until solid.
5. Break it up into big pieces after taking it out of the freezer. Serve immediately.

Nutrition: per serving

Calories: 196 kcal, 23 g of carbohydrates, 9 g of protein, 9 g of fat, 2 g of saturated fat, 2 g of polyunsaturated fat, 4 g of monounsaturated fat, 6 mg of cholesterol, 81 mg of sodium, 453 mg of potassium, 2 g of fiber, 19 g of sugar, 119 IU of vitamin A, 12 mg of vitamin C, 228 mg of calcium, 1 mg of iron.

Lemon Poppy Seed Cake

Ingredients

- All-purpose flour, 1/2 cup (325 g); 1 3/4 tsp baking powder
- One-fourth teaspoon baking soda
- Half a teaspoon of salt
- 1/2 cup (112 g) room-temperature unsalted butter
- 120 ml, or half a cup of veggie oil.
- 310g, or 1 1/2 cups, of sugar
- Half a teaspoon vanilla extract
- Four big eggs
- 180 ml, or 3/4 cup, of milk
- 120 ml, or half a cup, of fresh lemon juice
- Fresh lemon zest, two tablespoons
- Two tablespoons of poppy seeds
- Cream cheese with lemon frosting.
- 16 ounces (452 grams) room-temperature cream cheese

- 3/4 cup (172 g) of room-temperature butter
- Ten cups (1,150 grams) sugar powder
- Fresh lemon juice, 1 tablespoon.
- 1 tablespoon of fresh lemon juice

Instructions

1. Grease the edges of three 8-inch cake pans and line the bottom with circles of parchment paper. Set the oven temperature to 350°F (176°C).
2. In a larger basin, combine the flour, baking soda, baking powder, and salt; set aside.
3. In a large mixer bowl, combine the butter, oil, sugar, and vanilla extract. Beat for 1 1/2 to 2 minutes, or until the mixture is light in color and fluffy. Don't cut corners while screaming.
4. After each addition, stir the eggs until they are largely incorporated. To ensure that all of the ingredients are well combined, scrape down the bowl's sides as necessary.
5. Mix the batter until it is largely incorporated after adding half of the dry ingredients.
6. Slowly pour the milk and lemon juice into the batter and stir until well blended.
7. Mix in the remaining dry ingredients until smooth and thoroughly blended. To ensure that all of the ingredients are well combined, scrape down the bowl's sides as necessary. Avoid overmixing the batter.

8. Gently whisk together the poppy seeds and lemon zest.

9. Evenly distribute the mixture among the cake pans and bake for 22 to 25 minutes, or until a toothpick inserted into the center of the cake comes out with a few crumbs.

10. After taking the cakes out of the oven, let them cool for 2–3 minutes before transferring them to cooling racks to finish cooling.

11. To create the frosting, put the butter and cream cheese in a big bowl of a mixer and beat until creamy and thoroughly blended.

12. Add about half of the powdered sugar and stir until smooth and thoroughly blended.

13. Mix well after adding the lemon zest and juice.

14. Stir in the remaining powdered sugar until smooth and completely blended. For consistency, add as much or as little powdered sugar as you choose.

15. If necessary, use a broad serrated knife to flatten the domes on top of the cakes before assembling them.

16. Transfer the first cake to a cardboard cake ring or a serving plate.

17. Evenly cover the cake with roughly 1 cup of frosting.

18. Spread another cup of frosting over the second layer of cake.

19. Frost the outside of the cake and place the remaining layer on top. If necessary, see my guide on icing a smooth cake. I used one of the icing's ornamental sides to smooth out the line design on the cake's side.
20. Remove the cake as you see fit. I sprinkled some poppy seeds on top and put rosettes around the upper outside border. I also included several pieces of lemon.
21. Keep the cake chilled until it's time to serve. Although it's not always cold, cake tastes best when served chilled.

Nutrition: per-serving slice

Calories: 715 calories

94.3 g of sugar and 263.6 mg of sodium

26.7 g of fat,v115 g of carbohydrates, 7.5 g of protein

Pumpkin Spiced Oatmeal Cookies

Ingredients

- Two cups of all-purpose flour
- One and a half cups of uncooked, quick, or traditional oatmeal
- One teaspoon of baking soda
- One teaspoon of cinnamon

- Half a teaspoon of salt
- One cup of softened butter or margarine
- One cup of sugar
- One cup of packed brown sugar
- One cup of pumpkin pie filling (not canned pumpkin)
- One teaspoon of vanilla
- 3/4 cup of walnuts, chopped
- 3/4 cup of raisins
- One egg

Instructions

1. Turn the oven on to 350°F.
2. Apply nonstick cooking spray on cookie sheets.
3. Mix the flour, oatmeal, baking soda, salt, and cinnamon in a medium-sized bowl.
4. Beat the sugars and butter together in a large bowl until smooth and creamy.
5. Beat in the egg, pumpkin, and vanilla until well blended.
6. Add the dry ingredients gradually while pounding each time.
7. Add raisins and walnuts and stir.
8. Using a dough scoop or teaspoon, drop dough onto the cookie sheet.
9. Bake for 14–16 minutes, or until just beginning to brown.

10. After two minutes of cooling on the pan, transfer to a cooling rack.

Chocolate Banana Smoothie

Ingredients

- 1/4 cup plant-based or whey vanilla protein powder, 2 Tablespoons cocoa powder, 3/4 cup almond milk (or soy milk) ,1 medium frozen banana, 3–4 ice cubes

Instructions

1. Mix the milk, protein powder, and cocoa powder.
2. Add the ice cubes and frozen bananas.
3. Blend until smooth, enjoy!

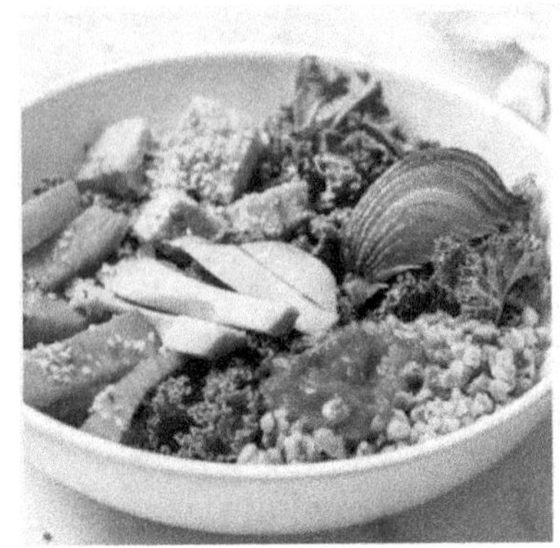
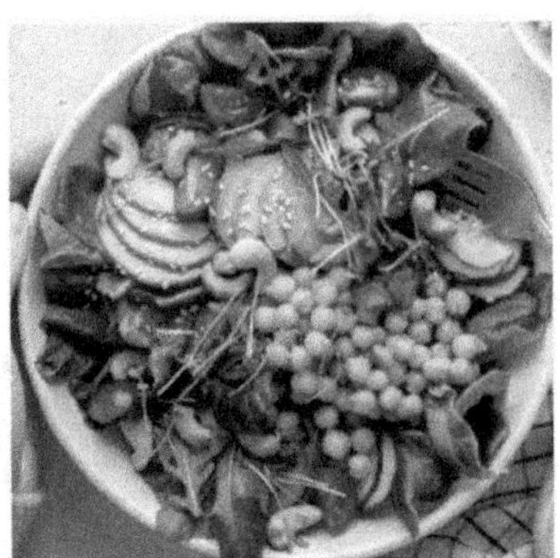

CHAPTER NINE

VEGETARAIN ANTI INFLAMMATORY DIET DELIGHTS

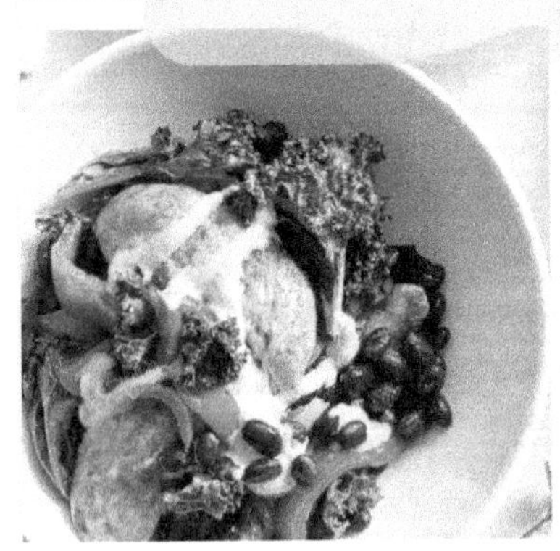
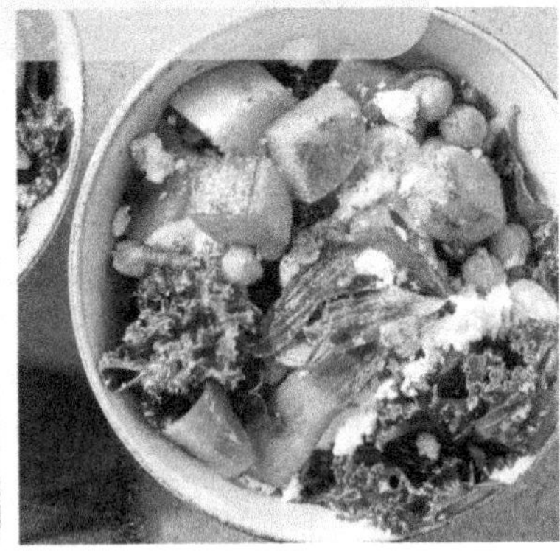

CHAPTER 9

VEGETARIAN AND VEGAN

Eggplant And Zucchini Lasagna

Ingredients

- One big eggplant, sliced into round or longitudinal slices that are 1/4 inch thick.
- Slice two or three big zucchini into rounds or lengthwise pieces that are 1/4 inch thick.
- 32 ounces of tomato sauce, around two cups
- Eight ounces of mozzarella cheese
- Two-thirds cup of parmesan cheese
- 1/4 cup chopped fresh basil
- One or two tablespoons of freshly chopped oregano and one or two teaspoons of olive oil.

Instructions

1. Set oven temperature to 425F.
2. Slice the eggplant and zucchini into 1/4-inch-thick slices, either in rounds or lengthwise into sheets, after removing the stems. Note: if cutting lengthwise, carefully use a

mandoline slicer; if cutting round, cut by hand with a knife.

3. To roast the veggies, grease two sheet pans, place the veggies on them, and bake them for 20 minutes.

4. After the eggplant and zucchini are cooked, add the lasagna in layers. Line the bottom of the baking dish with a thin layer of sauce, then add a layer of eggplant slices and a layer of zucchini. Finally, garnish with freshly chopped herbs and add mozzarella and parmesan cheese. Continue layering until all of the ingredients have been utilized.

Nutrition: per-serving

Calories: 147 kcal, 11.2 g of carbohydrates, 10.4 g of protein, 7.6 g of fat, 285.4 mg of sodium, 6.5 g of sugar, 11 IU of vitamin A, 20 mg of vitamin C.

Stir-fried Lentil And Vegetable Dish

Ingredients

- 1 tablespoon of oil
- 50g of shredded spring greens, one onion, one red pepper, and one halved and sliced courgette
- 400g container of washed and drained lentils
- Two tablespoons of sun-dried tomato paste.

- Wholewheat couscous, 100g

Instructions

1. In a frying pan, heat the oil and cook the veggies for four minutes. Cook for one minute after adding the lentils, tomato paste, and 100 milliliters of water. Adjust the seasoning to your preference.
2. In the meantime, put the couscous in a bowl, cover it with 200 milliliters of boiling water, and let it stand for five minutes. Serve the lentil and vegetable stir fry beside the couscous, which has been fluffed up with a fork.

Nutrition: per serving

Calories: 2,221 kJ/529 kcal of energy

20.8g of fat, 3.5g of saturated fat

65.9 g of carbohydrates, 15.4g of sugars

15.7g of fiber, 19.5g of protein, 1.3g of salt

Kebabs With Tofu And Vegetables

Ingredients

- 7 ounces of firm or extra-firm tofu;1 red bell pepper;1 red onion;2 cups of fresh pineapple.
- The marinade consists of two tablespoons of olive oil, one lime's juice, two garlic cloves, half a teaspoon each of smoked and sweet paprika, half a teaspoon each of curry powder, two teaspoons of BBQ sauce, and two tablespoons of water.

Instructions

1. Cut the tofu into cubes first.
2. After that, prepare the marinade. Put everything in a bowl and cover it. Give it a favorable toss.
3. Stir in the tofu cubes until the marinade coats them completely. Place the bowl in the refrigerator for at least two hours or overnight after covering it with the lid.
4. Make big chunks out of the pineapple.
5. Additionally, chop the red onion and bell pepper into big pieces.
6. Put everything together on wooden skewers. Start with a red onion and finish with it.
7. The skewers may be prepared on the stovetop or on the grill in a grilling pan. To ensure that the veggies and tofu are well browned, press them down several times with a spatula or barbecue tongs. Before serving, top them with finely chopped green onions and cilantro.

Nutrition: per-serving

Calories: 114 kcal, 12 g of carbohydrates, 4 g of protein, 6 g of fat, 1 g of saturated fat, 1 g of polyunsaturated fat, and 4 g of monounsaturated fat, 35 mg of sodium, 145 mg of potassium, 2 g of fiber, 8 g of sugar, 901 IU of vitamin A, 53 mg of vitamin C, 57 mg of calcium, and 1 mg of iron.

Curry With Chickpeas And Spinach

Ingredients

- Two tablespoons of olive or coconut oil, three crushed garlic cloves, one roughly chopped onion, one teaspoon paprika, half a teaspoon cayenne pepper, half a teaspoon ground coriander, a pinch of chili flakes, two tablespoons tomato puree, two cans of drained chickpeas, one vegetable stock cube or pot, 200 milliliters of water, one can of coconut milk, 60 grams of ground almonds, and 200 grams of spinach

Instructions

1. First, smash the garlic and chop the onion. Put the onion in a saucepan with oil over medium heat and cook for a few minutes until it softens.

2. Add the tomato puree and all the spices now, and stir.

3. Stir the ground almonds, coconut milk, vegetable stock, and drained chickpeas for five minutes over medium-high heat.

4. After removing the heat, toss in the spinach until it wilts.

Nutrition: per-serving

Calories: 480 kcal, 23g of carbohydrates, 15g of protein, 33g of fat, 2g of saturated fat, 12g of fiber, and 5g of sugar

Sweet Potato and Kale Hash

Ingredients

- 1 tablespoon olive oil, 1/2 cup diced red onion, 3 1/2 cups cubed and peeled sweet potatoes, 1 tablespoon minced garlic, 1 teaspoon each of salt, paprika, cumin, and black pepper, 3 cups finely chopped kale, 4 large eggs, 1/4 cup chopped cilantro for garnish, and 1 medium avocado

Instructions

1. In a skillet with heated olive oil, sauté the onion for about five minutes.

2. Sauté for a further minute after adding the garlic.

3. Add the sweet potato and spices, and simmer, covered, stirring every 5 minutes or so, until the potatoes are fork-tender—approximately 15 minutes.

4. Add the kale and cook for approximately two minutes, or until it has wilted.

5. Add the eggs to the hash after creating four wells. Cover and cook as desired.

6. Serve with avocado and toast and garnish with cilantro. Have fun!

Nutrition: per-serving

Calories: 348 kcal, 34 g of carbohydrates, 11 g of protein, 20 g of fat, 4 g of saturated fat, 3 g of polyunsaturated fat, 12 g of monounsaturated fat, 0.02 g of trans fat, 186 mg of cholesterol, 749 mg of sodium, 943 mg of potassium, 10 g of fiber, 7 g of sugar, 22125 IU of vitamin A, 57 mg of vitamin C, 213 mg of calcium, Iron: 3 mg.

Quinoa And Vegetable Stuffed Peppers

Ingredients

- Cut off the tops of six medium bell peppers and remove the cores. One cup of rinsed and drained uncooked quinoa, two cups of low-sodium vegetable broth, one tablespoon of olive oil, one small onion chopped, two minced garlic cloves, fifteen ounces of canned diced tomatoes, fifteen ounces of canned black beans, one cup of thawed frozen corn, one teaspoon each of cumin, paprika, salt, and black pepper, one cup of shredded Monterey Jack cheese, chopped cilantro, diced avocado, and sour cream (optional toppings)

Instructions

1. In a medium saucepan, combine the quinoa and vegetable broth. Over medium-high heat, bring the mixture to a boil. Reduce the heat to a simmer, place a lid on the pot, and cook for 15 minutes or until all of the liquid has been absorbed. Without lifting the cover, let the quinoa sit for about five minutes. Then, fluff it with a fork.

2. Cut the peppers in half lengthwise, remove the seeds and membrane, and preheat the oven to 375°F. When the peppers are cut side up, place them in a baking dish and fill the bottom of the pan with water.

3. In a large nonstick skillet, heat the olive oil over medium heat. Add the onions and cook for two to three minutes, or until they begin to soften. Cook for one more minute after adding the garlic until it becomes aromatic. Add the corn, black beans, chopped tomatoes, and cooked quinoa and stir.

Add salt, pepper, paprika, and cumin for seasoning. Cook for a further five minutes on low heat, stirring often.

4. Spoon the mixture into the pepper slices with care, then top with the cheese.
5. Bake uncovered for 30 to 35 minutes, or until the peppers are soft and the cheese has melted. Serve hot with optional toppings.

Nutrition: per-serving

Calories : 286 kcal, 51g of carbohydrates, 12g of protein, 5g of fat, and 1g of saturated fat per serving 915 mg of sodium, 907 mg of potassium, 12g of fiber, 8g of sugar, 4145 IU of vitamin A, 165 mg of vitamin C, 81 mg of calcium, and 4 mg of iron

Root Vegetables Roasted with Tahini Sauce

Ingredients:

*   root vegetables, totaling around 4 pounds; two beets, chopped and peeled; Two medium carrots, peeled and sliced on the bias, plus one or two big parsnipsOne big sweet potato, half an inch cubed; one large turnip, peeled and diced; one small yellow onion, chunked; one garlic bulb; one and a half cups of olive oil; one and a half teaspoons of kosher salt; one and a half teaspoons of freshly

ground black pepper; and two cups of chopped kale

The Tahini

- 1/3 cup tahini, 3 1/2 tablespoons olive oil, 1 1/2 tablespoons fresh lemon juice, 1 minced garlic clove, and 1/2 to 3/4 teaspoons fine sea salt are the dressing ingredients.To taste, freshly ground black pepper; ▫Two tablespoons chopped fresh parsley; two to three teaspoons honey; and five to six tablespoons of cool water
- Poached or soft-boiled eggs
- Parsley, chives, avocado, and walnuts

Instructions

1. Vegetables Roasted: Turn the oven on to 425°F. On a large baking sheet, combine the sweet potato, parsnips, carrots, turnips, onion, and beets with salt, pepper, and olive oil. Evenly distribute them across the pan.
2. Remove the garlic bulb's top and wrap it in a piece of foil. Cover with foil and drizzle with olive oil. The garlic foil package may be placed immediately on the oven rack or on the veggie pan.
3. For half an hour, roast the veggies. Check for soft garlic; if so, remove the package from the oven and set it aside. Return to the oven and roast for a

further 10 to 15 minutes after tossing the remaining veggies.

4. Add the chopped kale to the pan with the vegetables after they are fork-tender and have a hint of caramel. Squeeze the garlic cloves onto the baking sheet after removing them from the foil container. Mix everything together, then put it back in the hot oven for one to two minutes to allow the kale to wilt.

5. Dressing with Tahini: In the meanwhile, whisk together all of the dressing ingredients, except water. After combining them, gradually whisk in the cold water until the desired degree of creaminess is achieved. Continue whisking in more cold water until the dressing comes together if it seems to separate. Taste and adjust as necessary.

6. side view of a dish of roasted root veggies with an egg

7. Put together: Top the bowls with tahini dressing and the roasted veggies (or, if preferred, rice or quinoa). Add fresh herbs, a soft-boiled egg, and chopped walnuts as garnish.

Nutrition: per-serving
262 calories, 28.4 grams of carbohydrates, 5.5 grams of protein, 15.9 grams of fat, 5.7 grams of fiber, and 10.2 grams of sugar

Chickpea and Cauliflower Curry

Ingredients

- One red onion
- Four cloves of garlic
- One inch of ginger
- One tablespoon of medium curry powder
- One teaspoon of ground cumin
- Half a teaspoon of garam masala
- 1/4 teaspoon of turmeric powder
- 1/4 teaspoon powdered chili.
- 1/4 teaspoon of salt
- 400g of canned chopped tomatoes in one tin
- One tablespoon of tomato puree
- 400 ml of full-fat coconut milk in one tin
- 120 ml or half a cup of vegetable stock
- One medium cauliflower, or about four cups
- 400g of rinsed chickpeas and 1 tin
- Toppings are optional.
- A vegan cream drizzle
- Fresh coriander

Instructions

1. In a big pan, heat a tablespoon of oil over medium heat.
2. Let it simmer for a few minutes after adding the finely chopped onion. Next, add the grated ginger and minced garlic.
3. Stir to prevent burning; cook for one minute.

4. Curry powder, cumin, garam masala, turmeric, chili powder, and salt should all be added. Cook until aromatic, about 30 seconds. If it's too dry, add a little extra oil.

5. Add the tomato puree and diced tomatoes. Cook for a few minutes after stirring.

6. Transfer to a bowl, combine with a hand blender or in a blender until smooth, then put back in the pan.

7. Add the cauliflower, stock, and coconut milk. Don't cut the cauliflower into pieces that are too large or too little.

8. After 10 to 15 minutes of simmering, add the chickpeas and cook for an additional 5 minutes.

9. There should be some bite to the cauliflower, even if it is mushy. Cook it longer if you want it very tender.

10. Add some fresh coriander as a garnish and pour some vegan cream or coconut milk over it!

Nutrition: per-serving

Three servings

596 calories, 36 g of total fat, 27 g of saturated fat, 0g of trans fat, 6 g of unsaturated fat, 11 mg of cholestcrol, 181 mg of sodium, 57 g of carbohydrates, 17 g of fiber, 14 g of sugar, 20g of protein.

Sweet Potato Chili with Black Beans

Ingredients

- One tablespoon of olive oil
- One sliced onion
- Peel and cut two big sweet potatoes into ½-inch chunks.
- One chopped and seeded green bell pepper and four minced garlic cloves
- Two teaspoons of chili powder
- Two tablespoons of paprika
- Two teaspoons of cumin
- One teaspoon of oregano
- Half a teaspoon of black pepper and one teaspoon of salt
- Consume two cups of vegetable broth that is low in sodium.
- One 28-ounce can of fire-roasted chopped tomatoes with their liquids and two 15-ounce cans of rinsed and drained black beans
- One 4.5-ounce can of finely chopped green chilies and their juices
- Diced avocados for serving
- To serve, use fresh cilantro.

Instructions

1. Heat the olive oil in a big, heavy-bottomed saucepan over medium-high heat. Add the bell pepper, garlic, sweet potatoes, and onions. Stir to

mix, then simmer for 5 to 7 minutes, or until the veggies are tender and the onions are transparent.

2. To coat the veggies, add the chili powder, cumin, oregano, smoked paprika, salt, and pepper.
3. Add black beans, diced tomatoes and their juices, chopped green chilies and their juices, and vegetable broth. Bring the mixture to a boil after stirring it together.
4. To keep the pot simmering gently, cover it and lower the heat. Continue to cook for another 30 to 35 minutes, stirring occasionally, until the sauce thickens and the veggies continue to soften.
5. If preferred, top with fresh cilantro and chopped avocados after ladling into bowls.

Nutrition: per-serving

One serving

Calories 472 kcal, 90 g of carbohydrates, 19 g of protein, and 5 g of fat One gram of saturated fat, one gram of polyunsaturated fat, and three grams of monounsaturated fat 1994 mg of sodium, 1497 mg of potassium, 26 g of fiber, and 15 g of sugar 26772 IU of vitamin A, 51 mg of vitamin C, 245 mg of calcium, and 9 mg of iron.

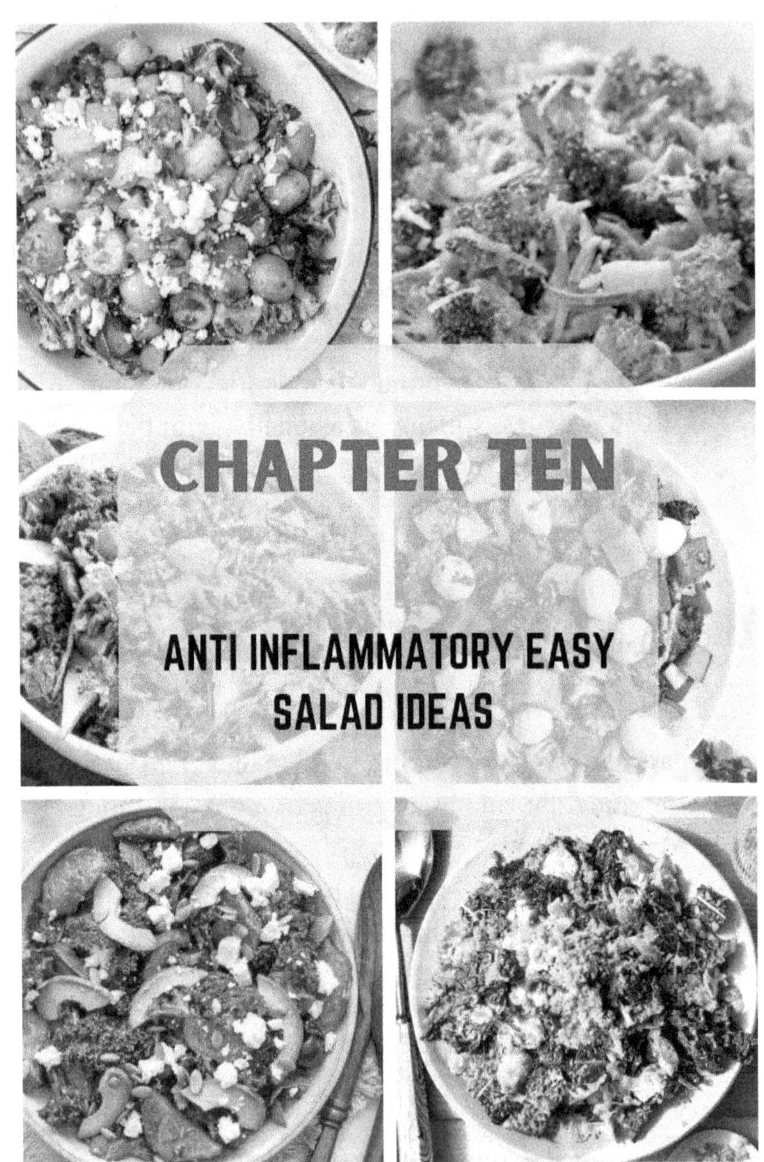

CHAPTER TEN

ANTI INFLAMMATORY EASY
SALAD IDEAS

CHAPTER 10

SALADS

Rainbow Salad With Turmeric Dressing

Ingredients

- Regarding the salads
- Six to eight cups of baby spinach
- 1 cup of cooked lentils (about 2 1/4 cups)
- One bunch of multicolored carrots
- Three medium beets, cut and peeled
- An additional 1 1/2 teaspoons of olive oil for tossing the spinach
- 1/4 teaspoon curry powder
- 1/4 teaspoon ground ginger
- A dash of cinnamon
- One fourth teaspoon of salt
- One-fourth teaspoon of pepper
- One avocado, cut into slices, a lemon squeeze, and hemp seeds as a garnish
- As a garnish, add sesame seeds.
- For garnish, use freshly chopped parsley.

Regarding the dressing

- 1/2 cup of one lemon's tahini juice

- 1 teaspoon ground turmeric and 1 1/2 tablespoons freshly grated ginger
- One spoonful of maple syrup, pure
- 1 teaspoon coconut aminos (which may be used instead of soy sauce)
- One fourth teaspoon of salt
- One-fourth teaspoon of pepper
- Half a cup of hot water

Instructions

1. Turn the oven on to 425°F. Put parchment paper on a big baking sheet with a rim. Place sliced beets and carrots on opposite sides of the sheet. Season with salt and pepper and drizzle with olive oil. Toss the carrots to coat them with curry powder, ground ginger, and cinnamon. Vegetables should be soft and brown after 25 to 30 minutes of roasting.
2. Bring a saucepan of water to a boil for the lentils in the meantime. Add a few pinches of salt to the water to season it. After it has boiled, add the lentils and simmer until they are cooked, about 20 minutes. Rinse with cold water after draining. Put aside.
3. Prepare the dressing. Whisk together the tahini, coconut aminos, maple syrup, ginger, turmeric, lemon juice, salt, and pepper. Whisk in the hot water until it's smooth and creamy.

4. Toss spinach in a big bowl, pour in some lemon juice, add salt and pepper to taste, and drizzle with olive oil. Toss to coat. Assemble the spinach by dividing it into bowls, then adding the roasted carrots and beets, sliced avocado, a drizzle of turmeric tahini sauce, a few spoonfuls of lentils, and a garnish of chopped parsley, sesame seeds, and hemp seeds.

Nutrition: per-serving

Four servings

578 calories, 28g of fat, 204 mg of sodium, and carbohydrates 60g, Sugar 15g, Protein 24g.

Caprese Salad with Balsamic Glaze

Ingredient

- Three vine-ripened or heirloom tomatoes, sliced into ¼-inch pieces
- Half a teaspoon each of sugar and salt, separated
- Slice one pound of fresh mozzarella into ¼-inch pieces (pre-sliced is OK).
- To taste, freshly ground black pepper
- Drizzling extra virgin olive oil.

- Store-bought balsamic glaze, a quarter cup of freshly chopped fresh basil, and additional entire sprigs to adorn the dish

Instructions

1. Slices of tomato should be arranged on a cutting board. After adding the sugar and ¼ teaspoon of salt, let it sit for a few minutes to allow the sugar to dissolve.
2. Place the mozzarella slices on a serving tray once the tomatoes have been cut. Evenly distribute the last ¼ teaspoon of salt and freshly ground black pepper on top. On top, drizzle a tablespoon of olive oil and the same amount of balsamic glaze (eyeball it). coarsely chopped basil. If desired, add fresh basil leaves to the plate as a garnish.

Nutrition: per serving

Six servings

264 calories, 19 g of fat, 10 g of saturated fat, 5 g of carbohydrates, 4 g of sugar, Fiber: 1 gram, 17 g of protein, Sodium: 672 mg, 60 mg of cholesterol.

Walnuts and Roasted Beets in a Spinach Salad

Ingredients

- Six beetroots (about two bunches), with the ends cut
- 60 milliliters (1/4 cup) One cup (100 g) of olive oil halves of walnuts
- 60 milliliters (1/4 cup) of vinegar made from red wine
- Freshly ground black pepper and salt
- 150g of baby spinach leaves per packet
- 100g of crumbled goat's cheese

Instructions

- First, preheat the oven to 200°C. The beets should be put on a baking pan. Bake in a preheated oven for one hour, or until a skewer inserted into the center comes out soft. Take it out of the oven and let it cool slightly for fifteen minutes. Peel the beets and cut it into wedges while wearing rubber gloves to prevent hand stains.
- Step 2: In the meantime, warm up the oil in a little skillet over medium heat. Toss in the walnuts and sauté for 2 to 3 minutes, or until they

are just beginning to toast. Take off the heat and let it cool.

- Step 3: Mix the walnut mixture with the vinegar. Season with salt and pepper after tasting.
- Step 4: Distribute the beets and young spinach leaves among the plates. Drizzle with walnut dressing and top with goat's cheese. Serve right away.

Nutrition: per-serving

Four servings

Calories:1289 kJ (308 cal) of energy

9.6g of protein, 26.5g of total fat, 6.5 g is saturated.

Total Carbohydrate: 10.7g, 5.9g of sugars, Sodium: 278.4 mg

Grilled chicken with Greek salad

Ingredients

- Six cups of chopped lettuce, such as romaine or iceberg
- One eight-oz Greek-marinated chicken breast, cut or sliced
- Two cups sliced tomatoes or a Mediterranean tomato salad

- One cup of hothouse or Persian cucumbers, sliced
- Half a cup of kalamata olives
- Half a cup of chunked feta cheese
- Regarding the Greek Dressing,
- ¼ cup red wine vinegar and extra virgin olive oil
- One clove of peeled and minced garlic
- Two tablespoons of oregano, dried
- One teaspoon of sugar and half a teaspoon of freshly ground black pepper and kosher salt

Instructions

1. Fill two separate salad bowls or a big serving dish with the lettuce. Add the cucumber, olives, feta cheese, tomato salad, and sliced chicken on top.
2. In a small canning jar, combine the olive oil, red wine vinegar, garlic, oregano, sugar, salt, and pepper to create the dressing. Place the lid on top and shake vigorously until fully combined and emulsified. To taste, add additional salt, pepper, and sugar.
3. Over the salad, drizzle the dressing and mix to taste.

Nutrition: per-serving

Calories: 334 kcal, 5g of carbohydrates, 3g of protein, 34g of fat, 7g of saturated fat, 17 mg of cholesterol, 476 mg of sodium, 25 mg of potassium, 1g of fiber, 3g of sugar, 180 IU of vitamin A, 0.5 mg of vitamin C, 133 mg of calcium, and 1.1 mg of iron per serving.

Lemon And Dill Salad With Tuna And White Beans

Ingredients

- One cup of washed and drained cannellini beans; five ounces of drained tuna in water; one teaspoon of lemon zest; one teaspoon of lemon juice; one clove of grated garlic; two teaspoons of extra virgin olive oil; one teaspoon of minced red onion; two tablespoons of fresh herbs (parsley, dill, basil, or mint); and salt and pepper to taste.

Instructions

1. In a medium bowl, combine the beans, tuna, onion, and fresh herbs.
2. Drizzle the bean mixture with olive oil, lemon zest, lemon juice, and garlic.
3. To taste, add salt and pepper. Serve on whole wheat toast, with crackers, or in lettuce cups.

Nutrition: per-serving

Calories: 230 kcal, 25 g of carbohydrates, 22 g of protein, 5.8 g of fat, 0.6 g of saturated fat, 32 mg of cholesterol, 588 mg of sodium, and 6.8 g of fiber

Mango And Shrimp Salad Dressed With Avocado

Ingredients

- 1 pound of big shrimp that have been deveined and skinned; 1 teaspoon of salt
- Half a teaspoon of powdered garlic
- Half a teaspoon of pepper
- Peel, pit, and chop two big mangoes into 1-inch pieces.
- Two big avocados that have been pitted, skinned, and sliced into 1-inch cubes
- Cut four Persian cucumbers into 1-inch cubes by halving them lengthwise.
- Peel and finely slice a small red onion.
- Regarding the Lime Honey Dressing
- Half a cup of newly extracted lime juice
- Two teaspoons of honey
- One tablespoon of olive oil, along with salt and pepper to suit.

Instructions

1. Put the shrimp, salt, pepper, and garlic powder in a bowl. Let it marinate for eight to ten minutes.
2. over a high temperature. Bring a grill pan that has been gently oiled to a high temperature. Cook the shrimp in a single layer for two to three minutes, or until they start to turn pink. Cook for another two to three minutes after turning.
3. Take out of the pan, cover, and refrigerate until fully chilled.
4. In the meantime, mix the olive oil, lime juice, honey, and salt & pepper to taste. Mix thoroughly.
5. Put the red onions, cucumbers, avocados, mangoes, and grilled shrimp in a big bowl.
6. Pour in the honey-lime dressing and mix gently.

Nutrition: per-serving

Four servings

Calories: 405 kcal, 34 g of carbohydrates, 26 g of protein, 20 g of fat, 2 g of saturated fat, 285 mg of cholesterol, 1473 mg of sodium, 836 mg of potassium, 8 g of fiber, 22 g of sugar, 1100 IU of vitamin A, 51.8 mg of vitamin C, 198 mg of calcium, and 3.3 mg of iron.

Goat Cheese, Strawberries, and Mixed Greens Salad

Ingredients

- 1 tablespoon of brown sugar or pure maple syrup
- Two teaspoons of vinegar from red wine
- Extra virgin olive oil, one tablespoon
- Half a teaspoon of salt
- To taste, freshly ground pepper
- Three cups of baby spinach
- Three cups of watercress with the stiff stems cut off
- Two and a half cups (12 ounces) of fresh strawberries, sliced
- ⅓ cup freshly chopped chives, sliced into pieces about 2 inches
- Half a cup of chopped toasted nuts and a quarter cup of crumbled goat cheese

Instructions

1. In a large bowl, whisk together maple syrup (or brown sugar), vinegar, oil, salt, and pepper. Toss to coat the spinach, lettuce, strawberries, and chives. Arrange the salad on four dishes and garnish with goat cheese and nuts.

Nutrition: per-serving

Four servings

Calories:206 kcal.

Dietary fiber (4g), total carbohydrates (15g), and added sugars (9g) 5g of protein (3g), 16g of total fat and 3g of saturated fat, 4 mg of cholesterol, 3212 IU of vitamin A, 81 mg of vitamin C, 79 mcg of folate, 218 mg of sodium, 101 mg of calcium, 2 mg of iron, 57 mg of magnesium, and 450 mg of potassium.

Watermelon And Feta Salad And Mints

Ingredients
- 2 tablespoons extra-virgin olive oil
- 3 tablespoons fresh lime juice
- ½ garlic clove, minced
- ¼ teaspoon sea salt
- 5 cups cubed watermelon
- Heaping 1 cup diced English cucumber
- ¼ cup thinly sliced red onion
- ⅓ cup crumbled feta cheese
- 1 avocado, cubed
- ⅓ cup torn fresh mint or basil leaves
- ½ jalapeño or serrano pepper, thinly sliced, optional
- Sea salt

Instructions

1. To make the dressing: In a small bowl, whisk together the olive oil, lime juice, garlic and salt.
2. Arrange the watermelon, cucumber, and red onions on a large plate or platter. Drizzle in half of the dressing. Top with the feta, avocado, mint, and serrano pepper, this is optional and drizzle with remaining dressing. Add salt to taste and serve.

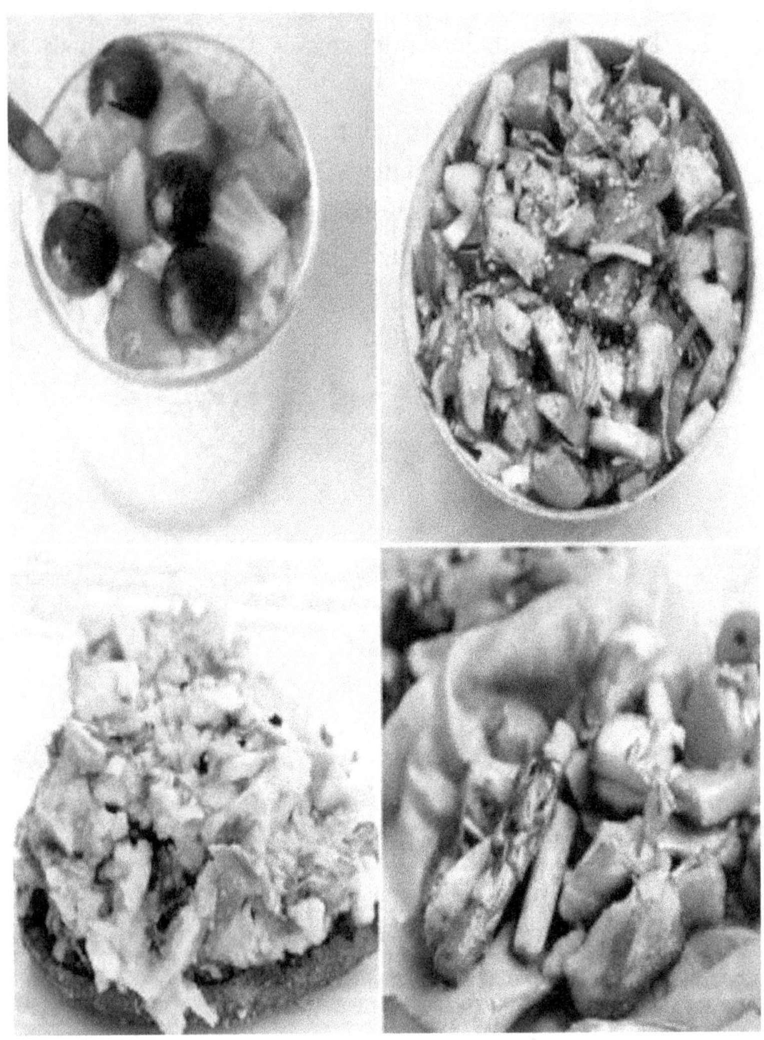

CONCLUSION

An anti-inflammatory diet is a long-term commitment to enhancing your general health and wellbeing, not a temporary solution. With the aid of ***Anti-Inflammatory Meal Plan,*** you may take charge of your diet in a sustainable manner, lowering inflammation and averting chronic illnesses before they start.

In addition to feeding your body, you're laying the groundwork for increased vitality, improved energy, and a more vibrant existence by adhering to the meal plans, using the meal prep advice, and implementing the delectable dishes into your everyday routine. This guide's steps are all intended to help you adopt a healthy lifestyle without feeling overburdened.

Keep in mind that every little adjustment matters as you go on your quest. In addition to improving your mood right now, an anti-inflammatory diet will have a significant long-term influence on your health. This book serves as a springboard—an encouragement to control your health by making dietary choices. Enjoy the meals, accept the process, and allow the healing to start.

Ultimately, leading an anti-inflammatory lifestyle involves more than simply avoiding certain foods; it also involves the foods you select to feed your body. You may easily and confidently make such healthy choices with the help of an ***Anti-Inflammatory Meal Plan***. Your path to improved health begins right now.